God of All Comfort

*A testimony of faith &
perseverance through infertility*

Written by
Kwenza Onyenakala

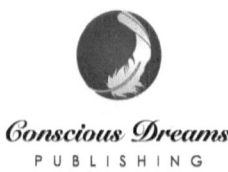

Conscious Dreams
PUBLISHING

Copyright © 2024: Kwenza Onyenakala.

All rights reserved. No part of this publication may be produced, distributed, or transmitted in any form or by any means, including photocopying, recording, or other electronic or mechanical methods, without the prior written permission of the publisher, except in the case of brief quotations embodied in critical reviews and certain other non-commercial uses permitted by copyright law.

Disclaimer

This book is a testimony of our faith. Even though the material within contains a lot of reference to medical science and procedures, it is in no way intended to be taken as medical advice. For expert knowledge and help with infertility, please consult with trained professionals.

Unless otherwise indicated, all Scripture quotations are taken from the New King James Version of the Bible.

First Printed in United Kingdom 2024

Published by Conscious Dreams Publishing
www.consciousdreamspublishing.com

Editor: Elise Abram

Cover Designer: Emily Rakic

Photo Credit: Eileen Bezuidenhout

Typesetter: Oksana Kosovan

ISBN: 978-1-915522-73-3

Dedication

To Afam.
The hero who is my husband and my best friend.
Thank you for loving me unconditionally and travelling this journey with me.

To every woman who has bravely faced the journey of infertility.
And to every couple that is still waiting…

*Blessed be the God and Father of our Lord Jesus Christ,
the Father of mercies and God of all comfort,
who comforts us in all our tribulation,
that we may be able to comfort those who are in
any trouble,
with the comfort with which we ourselves are
comforted by God.*
— 2 Corinthians 1:3-4

Contents

Dedication 3
Prologue 7
   Chapter I 9
   Chapter II 13
   Chapter III 21
   Chapter VI 31
   Chapter V 41
   Chapter VI 51
   Chapter VII 63
   Chapter VIII 75
   Chapter IX 83
   Chapter X 91
   Chapter XI 97
   Chapter XII 103
Motherhood Daily Declarations 107
About the Author 115
Acknowledgement 117
Works Cited 119

Prologue

THE SUN IS SETTING AS my husband, and I take a walk on the pebbled beach in Kent. We're holding hands and headed for a certain familiar spot where we sit down. It has been a lovely day, and we both feel relaxed in the scorching sun. Even though the sun is cooling down, I am careful to keep on my sun hat to protect against sun damage. I was exposed to the harsh African sun from a young age, but my skin is not as tolerant now. I look around, admiring the beautiful beach mansions, as we compare which one is our favourite. The tide has gone out, leaving all manner of small sea life exposed. The seagulls are calling out to each other in the distance, and we hear the laughter of children playing in the water on the other side of the beach. I am bursting with happiness today, but I remember a scenario that unfolded this time last year in the same spot when everything was different. As I take my husband's hand and deeply inhale the fresh smell of the sea, I remember having taken his hand at that time, saying the words I had been dreading for a long time. I remember breaking down in tears even before I could finish those words, my heart broken into little pieces…

CHAPTER 1

*Now faith is the substance of things hoped for, the evidence
of things not seen.
For by it the elders obtained a good testimony.*
— Hebrews 11:1-2

It was going to be a good day; I could feel it in my spirit. You do that when you're a Christian woman who has re-dedicated her life to serving Christ, and you feel the move of God as you walk into church on a Sunday morning. Dressed as you envisioned yourself when you bought the outfit you're wearing, you know you'll turn a few heads and get a few comments about how well your dress works with your heels. I caught my reflection in the glass doors leading to the foyer and liked what I had seen. I had a light spring to my step and a big smile on my face.

My bestie was already inside, and I made my way over to where she was sitting. The worship team had started to drum away, and I was getting in the mood to sing and worship. I love God, and I love the buzz of a Sunday morning at church, and there was no other place I'd rather have been on that day. I was not serving on any of my teams that morning, and I looked forward to dedicating all my attention to the worship service and soaking in the sermon my pastor would preach afterwards. My notebook and pen were ready in my matching handbag. It took me a while to get used to using the notepad on my phone to take notes in church. It somehow felt wrong, but I do it nowadays. After all, is it not God who created the intelligence of man that enabled us to invent modern technology? I still prefer the hard copy of my Bible though, compared to the downloadable version.

I kept on walking, stopping now and again for a brief chit-chat with different people as you do on a Sunday morning, mostly about how the week had been. I gave a fluttering little wave here and there and whispered "Hi" to those in the distance. You don't just walk straight to your seat on a Sunday morning. You acknowledge the others and make a show of noticing new faces and making them feel welcome. If you are a member of the serving teams, your hospitality does not end on your serving day.

I finally got to my seat, and my bestie stood up to make way for me to sit — as she had gotten there first, she had taken the aisle seat. After the usual hugs, air kisses, and exclamations of "Girl, I missed you this week," we sat down. We soon stood when the first worship song was played, and I lifted my hands, ready to worship my God.

I was getting ready to close my eyes to worship when I saw him. He walked into the auditorium wearing a sharp black suit and a white shirt. Good thing I hadn't closed my eyes yet! I lowered my hands, stared, swallowed and smiled, my heart racing. It was then that I heard that still small voice in my head or my heart, I don't remember which. It must have been both. The voice said, "I'm going to marry that man." Yes, it was going to be a good day after all!

Such confidence. Such faith. The Cambridge English Dictionary defines confidence as "a feeling of little doubt about yourself and your abilities or feeling of trust in someone or something." When writing about faith, Capps, author of *Faith and Confession*, says that "true faith is never blind. Faith always knows. Faith always sees. Faith is able [sic] to look through the storm and see the end results" (19). I couldn't agree more.

I don't know if it was my confidence or my faith that propelled me to do what I did next and in the next coming weeks. Whatever it was, it paid off because after dating for nearly two years from that day, we got married in sunny Cape Town in what most of our family and friends still think was the wedding of that year. It was 2015, and I celebrated my 39th birthday on our honeymoon that year.

CHAPTER II

There is no fear in love;
but perfect love casts out fear because fear involves torment.
But he who fears has not been made perfect in love.
— 1 John 4:18

YES, MY FAIRY TALE HAD BEGUN. It was the fairy tale I had prayed for, worshipped, and praised God for. He had given me exactly what I had asked for when I had gone on my knees and said, "Lord, I am not a hunter. I will worship You and praise You and when the time is right, You will bring the right man into my life." God had given me a man who looked into my eyes with all my imperfections and told me that I was God's daughter. In God's eyes I was perfect, and when he looked at me, he had seen perfection, a man who reminded me of God's perfect love that casts out all fear. For you see, with all my confidence and faith, I had a hidden fear, one from the past, that the enemy dangled in front of me at every opportunity. It was a past with the profound potential to stir up my marriage, depending on how it was handled.

The word *fear* is a broad term that can be explained in different ways and is specific to the context in which it is described. I like the Cambridge English Dictionary version, which says it is "a strong emotion caused by great worry about something dangerous, painful or bad that is happening or might happen." Whether it is an immediate response or a long-term response, fear brings about different emotions and reactions for different people depending on the situation. Fight or flight is a common reaction in immediate situations of danger. My fear was a long-term one, and one of the emotions it brought with it was self-doubt.

Years ago, I had lain in a hospital bed, listening with disbelief as an obstetric surgeon looked at me with sorrow in his eyes and told me that he had regretfully failed to save my second fallopian tube. My other fallopian tube, the right one, had been removed three months earlier. Unfortunately, as he continued to explain, this meant I could not be expected to conceive naturally ever again. I already had one child, but I had fallen pregnant twice since then, and both times the pregnancy had been ectopic.

Ectopic pregnancies occur when the fertilised egg does not make it to the womb cavity but instead implants itself in the fallopian tube. As the embryo grows, the tube cannot handle the pressure, and in most cases, it ruptures. Ectopic pregnancies are obstetric emergencies requiring immediate surgery. Doctors try to save the fallopian tube, but in most the cases, this is not possible, and they are forced to remove the tube in what is medically termed a salpingectomy. In most cases, when women experience an ectopic pregnancy, it leaves them with one fallopian tube with which to conceive in the future, but I had lost both.

I listened with mixed feelings as my obstetric surgeon told me that my case was one in a million that he had not yet come across in his long-standing career. Though I was shocked, I was grateful that in both cases, I had the best medical attention. Nonetheless, I found myself asking God why. Why me? Why now? What had I done wrong to deserve this? Strangely enough, I don't remember crying much. It was a different time; I was in a different marriage, and I concluded that it was God's way of getting me out of a difficult situation, as my marriage ended not long after that.

A lot of things happen to a lot of people that are unexplainable, and we are left wondering and asking God why, but He is the God of our past, present and future. The Bible says, "For you formed my inward parts; you covered me in my mother's womb" (Ps. 139:13). This tells us that God knows us from the beginning, and He knows where we are headed. God continues to reassure us of this when He says, "See, I have inscribed you on the palm of my hands" (Isa. 49:16).

I have always known God throughout my life. Though at the time, I did not have a deeper, intimate relationship with Him, God is always engaged in an intimate relationship with us regardless of where we are in life or what we might be going through. He is there to protect us and save us, as He did with me during my two medical emergencies. God's plans are always good for us: "For I know the thoughts that I think toward you, says the Lord, thoughts of peace and not of evil, to give you a future and a hope" (Jer. 29:11).

I think that sometimes, the enemy, or the devil, steals God's script and peeks at what God has written about us. He then throws giants and weeds in our path, so it takes us longer to reach our destinations and fulfil God's promises. Why does God let this happen? So that we can grow in our faith and learn to trust Him through it all. The Bible reminds us of how God works everything out for our good (Rom. 8:28). Most people would agree that this is not easy to understand in times of suffering, but God is an ever-present God, who is always with us in the storm. This reminds me of a time in the Gospel of John when Jesus healed a blind man. Before healing him, the disciples asked Jesus who had sinned between the man and his parents such that he was born blind. Jesus answered, "Neither this man nor his parents sinned, but that the works of God should be revealed in him" (John 9:3). Some situations happen so that God may be glorified through His miraculous ways. The only challenge is understanding this when unpleasant situations happen.

I had moved on with life, but the enemy had given me a new identity with which to describe myself. My new identity was as a woman who could no longer bear children. One of my pastors has preached about how a lot of people find themselves with new identities in life: divorcee, recovering drug addict, jailbird, and so on. The enemy does a victory dance when we are held captive by these identities because it means we cannot move on to experience the full life God has in store for us. He encourages people not to allow the enemy this victory by saying, "The enemy will show you ashes… but God says I'm going to give you beauty for the ashes" (Norman 1:43:35) and "Don't let one negative event become your identity" (Norman 1:34:10). I had lived in my captivity for a long time.

That is, until God brought my king into my life. In the days when we were dating and getting to know each other, the enemy poked me with my fear numerous times. Those feelings of self-doubt crept up now and again: my king had not fathered a child yet — was I the right woman to take on this task? Would I ever have the joy of holding another child in my arms? What if it didn't happen? What would it mean for our marriage?

Self-doubt is the destroyer of dreams and aspirations. It says that you can't, it's not possible, it's not for people like you. It is the thing that stops us from reaching our potential and letting go of God's promises. Self-doubt makes one only see giants. It takes a strong will and mentality to fight it. It is what I would like to call a 'Caleb mentality'.

In the Bible story of the Exodus of the children of Israel, Moses sent twelve spies into the land of Canaan to assess if they could infiltrate the land as promised by God. This was after the children of Israel had been delivered from bondage in Egypt, and God had led them through the wilderness to the border of Canaan (Num. 13:1-33). Some of the spies brought back a bad report, saying that the people were giants, and they were strong, and Israel would surely lose the battle if they tried to conquer it. It was Caleb, one of the spies, who said, "Let us go up at once and take possession, for we are well able to overcome it" (Num. 13:30). He knew that God had already given them the land and would make a way. It takes a great deal of discernment to know that this thought, idea, or situation has been planted by God. One's confidence to go for things might be shaken, but God is well and able to make a way.

Even though the enemy kept throwing the emotion of self-doubt my way, the woman he had attacked so many years ago was not the same woman today. I was in a better place, stronger and not easily intimidated. I knew about putting on the armor [sic] of God to fight my battles, and I recognised what had happened to me so long ago for what it was: an attack by the principalities of darkness on a woman at a young age. The Apostle Paul reminds us of this when he says:

> *Put on the whole armor of God, that you may be able to stand against the wiles of the devil. For we do not wrestle against flesh and blood, but against principalities, against powers, against the rulers of the darkness of this age, against spiritual hosts of wickedness in the heavenly places. Therefore, take up the whole armor of God, that you may be able to withstand in the evil day, and having done all, to stand* (Eph. 6:11-13).

I was determined not to cower. God was still writing my story, and I trusted Him. He had opened a door I thought had been shut the day the doctor had given me my medical prognosis. For so long, the enemy made me believe that I would never be good enough for any man as I could not produce offspring for them, but God had given me back my confidence. He promised me that He was the one who went before me, He would be with me, He would neither leave me nor forsake me, and I should neither fear nor be dismayed (Deut. 31:8). He constantly reminded me of His peace that surpassed all understanding and guided my heart and my mind (Phil. 4:6-7), and that no weapon formed against me would prosper (Isa. 54:17). Armed with this knowledge, I put my feelings of doubt aside and bravely faced the future.

CHAPTER III

Behold children are a heritage from the Lord, The fruit of the womb a reward.
Like arrows in the hand of a warrior, so are the children of one's youth.
Happy is the man who has his quiver full of them; They shall not be ashamed but shall speak with their enemies in the gate.
— Psalm 127:3-5

LIKE ANY NEWLY MARRIED COUPLE, after the giddiness of the honeymoon period comes the settling down and then the inevitable baby planning. Our Christian faith reminds us that we serve a God of miracles, so we believed that God had the ability to perform a natural conception even after what the doctors had said in the past. There was always the hope at the back of my mind that maybe the doctors had made a mistake and one of my fallopian tubes would miraculously repair itself one day. After trying for a while, we knew we could not avoid the inevitable, and we had to seek medical attention as we were facing infertility.

On their 'Infertility' page, The World Health Organisation (WHO) explains that "infertility is a disease of the male or female reproductive system, defined by the failure to achieve a pregnancy after 12 months or more of regular unprotected sexual intercourse." According to the National Health Service (NHS) statistics, infertility is believed to affect 1:7 heterosexual couples in the United Kingdom alone ("Overview: Infertility"). They go on to explain that there are two types of infertility: primary and secondary. Primary being when one has never conceived before and the latter, when one is having difficulty getting pregnant again. If I were to put myself in a category, I would say I had secondary infertility as I already had one child.

The decision to seek medical attention can be difficult because most people don't know how long waiting 'long enough' is. On the same page, the NHS advises that people should seek treatment if they have not conceived after a year of trying. For Christian couples, this can be even more challenging because we believe in God's timing. "To everything there is a season, A time for every purpose under heaven" (Eccl. 3:1). We may feel that when seeking medical help, we doubt God and are not exercising our faith properly or trying to help God.

Conception is a process involving both male and female reproductive systems. The anatomy of the female reproductive system is comprised of the vulva, the vagina, the cervix, the uterus, the fallopian tubes and the ovaries, all of which are supported by ligaments in the pelvis. The male reproductive system includes the penis, scrotum, testicles, vas deferens, prostate and urethra. There are also some key reproductive hormones involved in both male and female reproductive systems. Any book on anatomy and physiology can give this information in more detail.

For uncomplicated conception to take place, all the systems, from the hormones to the organs, should be in healthy order. There are many risk factors and medical conditions that can affect any part of the reproductive system for either males or females. Seeking medical assistance can prompt a medical examination that will pick up any areas of the system that have been negatively affected. Doctors can then intervene with corrective procedures and treatments. Some conditions can be more challenging to treat than others. In some cases, doctors may recommend assisted reproduction therapies (ART). For those from a Christian faith background, knowing where the enemy has attacked is helpful, as prayer can be made more specific and focused around that area.

Female infertility is a condition that has affected women since time immemorial. Across history, whether it's biblical or cultural, a couple's failure to conceive is usually viewed as being down to the female. This perspective has changed in modern times as more research is done to explore the factor of male infertility, but this does not rule out the fact that the burden of productivity almost always relies on the female partner. Little girls still play with dolls from a young age and grow up expecting to have a baby of their own one day.

In humanity, marriage and children go hand in hand. The Bible says when God created man, he said, "Be fruitful and multiply; fill the earth and subdue it" (Gen. 1:28). Children are perceived to complete a marriage unless the couple have decided they do not want to have children. In some societies, a man's virility is measured by the number of children he has produced. In the Bible children are likened to arrows, and the man whose quiver (a case for arrows) is full of them is not ashamed (Ps. 127:4). My understanding of this scripture is that children are perceived as a weapon, and a man with children can stand up in dignity amongst other men. Such perspectives add a lot of pressure on women struggling to conceive.

In today's world, women can choose to have children without getting married and sometimes end up not getting married to the fathers of their children due to different circumstances. Whatever the situation, it cannot be denied that the drive for most women to conceive and bear a child is an inborn instinct.

It is this that drove even great women of the Bible to take matters into their own hands. In the book of Genesis, God made a promise to Abram (name later changed to Abraham) that he would be a father of many nations (Gen. 15:1-6). As time went on and they got on in years, Sarai (name later changed to Sarah), his wife, could not see how this was going to happen as she was barren (the biblical term for being infertile). She then offered her maidservant, Hagar, to Abraham to bear them an heir, thinking this would fulfil God's plans (Gen. 16:2-6). More than that, I think Sarah thought it would fill the hollow feeling she had felt for so long at not being able to hold her husband's child. However, this arrangement did nothing to appease that desire. Contrary to what she had envisioned, it would have hurt her deeply to watch Abraham decorating the nursery with Hagar while embracing her and stroking her blossoming abdomen as they awaited the birth of the child. I imagine Sarah watching Abraham and Hagar while thinking, 'that should be me.'

Ishmael was born to Hagar, but Sarah failed to embrace the child as Hagar looked down upon Sarah for not being able to conceive. God finally visited Sarah at the appointed time, and she gave birth to Isaac. At Isaac's weaning party, Sarah asked Abraham to expel Hagar and Ishmael from the land. She and Hagar could not get along as Sarah felt that their biological son, Isaac, was Abraham's rightful heir (Gen. 21:1-21). This situation had a profound impact on the course of Biblical history, and it all began with one woman's desire to produce an heir for her husband. It is this same desire that is embedded in so many women's hearts.

The twelve tribes of Israel, as they are known today, originated from the battle between two sisters to produce children for their husband, Jacob. Rachel, who was loved by her husband, could not conceive, and ended up giving her maidservant to Jacob to bear children for her. Having been given to Jacob because of her father's treachery, Leah was not loved by Jacob (Gen. 29:21-30), but God had blessed her womb. She kept having children, hoping that her husband would love her after each pregnancy. This did not happen, as Jacob still only had eyes for the childless Rachel, which added to Leah's frustration. Leah even went so far as to give her maidservant to Jacob in a bid to outdo Rachel when it came to baby-making, hoping he would love her more. This shows that for most women, the ability to have children is almost always attached to the desire to be loved, respected, and approved of. God finally visited Rachel and gave her Joseph, who became Jacob's favourite son as he was born out of love (Gen. 29:1-35; 30:1-24).

In the later chapters of the Bible, we meet Hannah and Peninnah, who were married to Elkanah. Hannah had no children, but she was loved more by her husband. Elkanah could not understand why Hannah was sad all the time as he did his best to show his love even though she had not borne him any children. He would ask, "Hannah why do you weep? Why do you not eat? And why is your heart grieved? Am I not better to you than ten sons?" (1 Sam. 1:8), but Hannah's desire to produce a child for her husband was so deep that her husband's love could not replace it. Her marriage did not feel complete and her rival, Peninnah, always mocked her for being childless. I can only picture Hannah's anguish as she visited the well to collect water, meeting all the women with their children while her rival took the opportunity to mock and laugh at her.

There is an unspoken approval in society for women who bear children, and Hannah needed to bear a child to gain that respect as a woman. So, Hannah heads to the temple to pray "in bitterness of soul and weeping in anguish" until she appears like a drunk woman to the Priest Eli who reassures her to go in peace as God will grant her request (1 Sam. 1:17). God finally heard her cry and gave her Samuel, whose life she dedicated to the Lord, and he went to live in a temple. She had made a deal with God while praying in the days before he was conceived, and she would not have the joy to see him grow every day, nor would she be able to guide him through his milestones, but glory be to God! Let it be known that Hannah finally conceived and bore a child for her husband, and God blessed her with even more children as she had honoured her promise.

When Rachel conceived and bore a son for Jacob, she said, "God has taken away my reproach" (Gen. 30:23). God likens the nation of Israel to a barren woman when referring to its restoration and says, "Do not fear, for you will not be ashamed; Neither be disgraced for you will not be put to shame" (Isa. 54:4). When Elizabeth gave birth to John the Baptist after many years of barrenness, she expressed how God had taken away her reproach among people (Luke 1:25). In this context, the word 'reproach' refers to disapproval or disappointment.

This same stigma and sense of shame is still expressed by women today as the social and cultural consequences of the failure to conceive bear resemblance across the globe. Noni Martins is a Zimbabwean-British Blogger whose Blog Unfertility.com offers a diversity lens and nuance to the discussion of infertility. She has shared her infertility journey from a cultural perspective. She states how the music was still playing at her wedding when people started to ask when they intended to start a family. In her cultural upbringing, the talk was always about fertility and never infertility. She goes on to say, "The reality is that as a black woman, to accept (what I now know to be infertility) is to have your womanhood invalidated. I know this is not true because I am an enlightened millennial, but it can feel this way" (Martins). She mentions hearing stories of women being sent back to their families if they couldn't bear children.

Indeed, across the Sub-Saharan African region women who have failed to conceive have been known to face: "marital instability and divorce, domestic abuse, polygamy, stigmatisation by the family and community, social isolation, accusations of witchcraft, limited rights to land and financial inheritance" (Elwell). Some of this treatment stems from traditional practices such as the Lobola bride price (also known in other terms in different regions). This practice which is common in my own culture requires the groom's family to pay a price to the bride's family in the form of livestock or money. This is to symbolize that the children born of the union will legally belong to the husband's lineage. If a woman has failed to fall pregnant it means that they are not able to meet the demands of this contract.

Authors Lamb and Adegbile's collection of stories highlights some struggles faced by women from a Black, Asian, and ethnic minority background in the United Kingdom. Some of the stories show the unforgiving nature of some cultures, which can drive women to heartbreaking and almost unsafe lengths to mother children for their husbands. In the wider cultural context, Logan et al., describe how in Chinese culture childlessness is often perceived as the woman's fault and how infertile women are highly stigmatised. In some Muslim communities' children are regarded as a source of income and security in old age. There is also a preference of sons over daughters as sons will carry on the family name in this community (Ali et al.). In Northern Vietnam being fertile is highly favoured as generational continuity is tied to deep rooted beliefs such as ancestral worship and a connection of the living to the dead (Pashigan). This ancestral connection is also valued in Middle Eastern cultures (van Rooij et al.) and in Chinese culture (Logan et al.).

Most countries ruled by monarchs thrive on the production of heirs to the throne. In "Royal Succession," the History.com editors mention some factors that have affected smooth succession in some monarchies. They observed that "the inability of some monarchs to produce a suitable male heir has resulted in confusion and tumultuous transfers in power." Some business empires rely on the offspring to carry on and keep the family business in the bloodline. When children are not produced, it can leave a trail of power struggles threatening to tear family legacies apart.

In comparison, Western societies are more forgiving in that it is socially acceptable for couples to decide not to have children. Having children through surrogacy or donated gametes (eggs and sperm) is also more acceptable in Western culture than in other cultures. Still, women struggling to conceive in this society can face the same emotional struggles and stigmas. The website IVFBabble.

com is an online fertility and IVF resource where people going through infertility can join the community and share their stories. Caucasian women predominantly engage on this platform and some of the stories they share can be quite moving.

Up until that point, I had not experienced any kind of pressure from my husband or his family and even our social circle. There was the odd person who would ask, but most people kept a respectable distance and didn't talk about it. At the start of our relationship, my husband reassured me that he would love me the same even if we did not have children. Our happiness together was more important. Nonetheless, this reassurance did nothing to stop my heart's desire to have his children. Besides wanting to carry a child for him out of my love and respect, my feelings were also influenced by my own African culture and traditional upbringing. In my culture, women must be fertile and produce children. Although we didn't talk at length about this, I was sure that his being a British man of Black African descent, the expectations were the same in his culture. I told myself that I had to carry a child for my husband for his legacy to carry on, out of my desire to feel as if our marriage was complete and for his dignity as a man in society. My son from my first marriage was now in his twenties and had flown the nest. I felt that I needed to fill the nest with my husband's offspring and wear my crown in his family. I needed God now more than ever.

CHAPTER IV

So, God created man in His own image; in the image of God He created him; male and female He created them.
— **Genesis 1:27**

WHEN WE DECIDED TO SEEK medical attention, it was towards the end of 2016, when I was 40 years old. The first point of call was our GP. By then, we had figured out that we would need in vitro fertilisation (IVF) to conceive. I was living in Zimbabwe when my fallopian tubes were removed. IVF was not a common procedure in my country, and the doctor who had performed my surgery did not mention it as an option. I don't blame him. There were no IVF facilities in my country, so discussing it would have been irrelevant. My husband and I had touched on it at the start of our relationship. I knew about IVF from my own medical knowledge as a nurse. What I didn't know was all the finer details of the process.

IVF is one of the few procedures used in assisted reproductive technology (ART). In its online glossary, the UK government fertility regulator, the HFEA, explains that this is when fertilisation takes place outside the body ("In vitro fertilisation (IVF)"). In summary, a treatment cycle involves suppressing natural hormone production, followed by hormone treatment to boost egg supply. Then, the eggs are collected and mixed with the sperm to fertilise and produce embryos. This is followed by embryo transfer into the womb. It sounded simple enough, and I was excited at the prospect of being able to show off my baby bump sometime soon.

Since the first 'test tube baby', Louise Brown, was born in 1978, IVF treatment has made it possible for many families struggling with infertility to conceive and experience parenthood. Like many other medical procedures that have either saved or changed lives, IVF is one of medical science's major breakthroughs of the century. Even though this procedure has given hope to couples struggling to conceive, there is never a guarantee it will work. It also comes with its medical challenges and adverse reactions such as ovarian hyperstimulation syndrome (OHSS) and in some cases, cycles must be cancelled, and the couple loses money. An expensive procedure that is unavailable in countries with low income, IVF can also take its toll on those who must go through cycle after cycle in the hope of getting pregnant. Conversely, when it works, IVF brings families much joy and completeness.

It has also been subjected to much scepticism due to the ethical implications attached. Many have critiqued the use of IVF to form life. The continuous innovation of this procedure and the varying combinations through which family units can be achieved through IVF make some even more critical of this area of medicine. This observation was also documented many years ago by Strong. In his book, Strong states how "scientific advances in reproductive and perinatal medicine are producing a bewildering array of ethical questions" (3). On their page, The Ethics Centre reiterate these misgivings by saying:

> *Some people object to the artificial creation of a life that would not be possible if left entirely to nature. Or they might object on the grounds that 'natural selection' should be left to do its work. Others object to conception being placed in the hands of mortals rather than left to [sic] God* ("The Ethics of In Vitro Fertilization").

Some of these concerns stem from the fact that couples sometimes have good success and end up with better-quality embryos than can be transferred into the womb. Some embryos end up not being needed, depending on the number of children for which the couple had planned. It is the fate of these embryos to end up either being used for research purposes, frozen for future use, donated to other couples or destroyed.

This poses many ethical questions as it can be argued that an embryo is a life formed. No human has the right to take another human's life or make flippant decisions about their welfare. Those seeking answers might find themselves asking questions such as whether the word embryo is an umbrella term for stages in pregnancy development. Is an embryo a 'life formed' or a 'life in formation'? To answer these questions, one must delve deeper into the science of embryonic development. I found a detailed account of this in Biga et al.'s *Oregon State University Anatomy and Physiology*. The authors explain that "the first 2 [sic] weeks of prenatal development are referred to as the pre-embryonic stage. A developing human is referred to as an embryo during weeks 3–8 [sic], and a foetus from the ninth week of gestation until birth."

Fertilisation between the egg (also referred to as an oocyte) and the sperm takes place in the fallopian tubes. The fertilised egg is called a zygote and it contains all the genetic material from the mother and the father which is needed to form a human. At this stage, the zygote undergoes rapid cell division from two cells to four cells to eight cells while in the fallopian tube. It then reaches the uterus in its 16-cell stage division and is now called a morula by Day 3 ("Week 3"). Cell division continues for the next few days to 70–100 cells, forming what is called a blastocyst ("What is the difference"). Within the blastocyst, the inner group of cells will become the embryo, and the outer layer will give rise to part of the placenta.

The pre-embryonic stage of development ends when the blastocyst embeds itself in the uterine lining to begin the process of implantation ("28.2. Embryonic Development"). The following images clarify this process further.

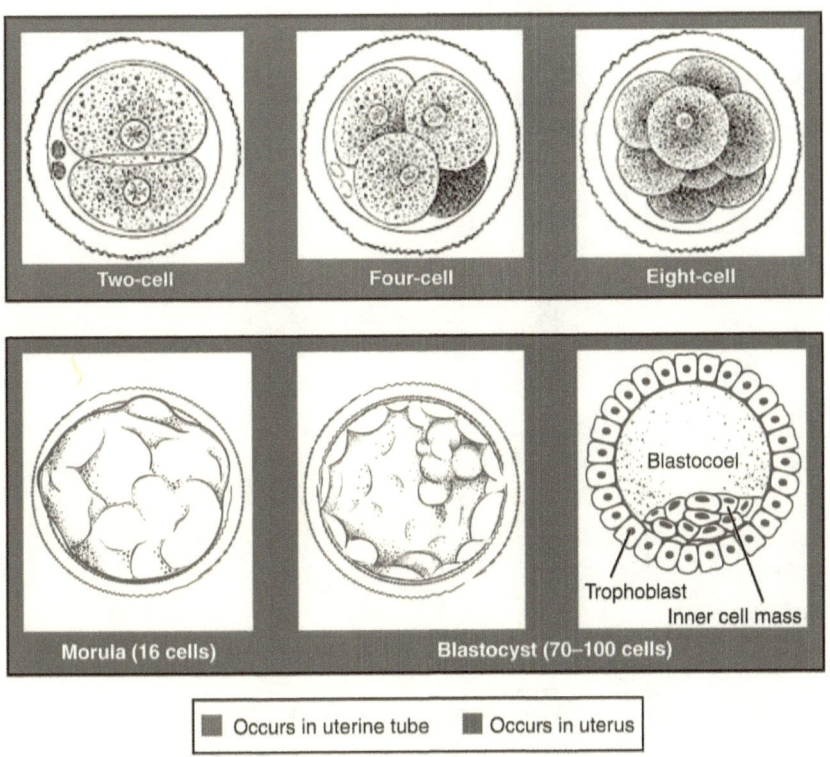

Figure 28.2.1[1]**—Pre-Embryonic Cleavages:** Pre-embryonic cleavages make use of the abundant cytoplasm of the conceptus as the cells rapidly divide without changing the total volume (Biga et al. 28.2).

---

1 *Images, from Anatomy & Physiology by OpenStax, are licensed under CC BY except where otherwise noted. CC BY 4.0 Deed | Attribution 4.0 International | Creative Commons*

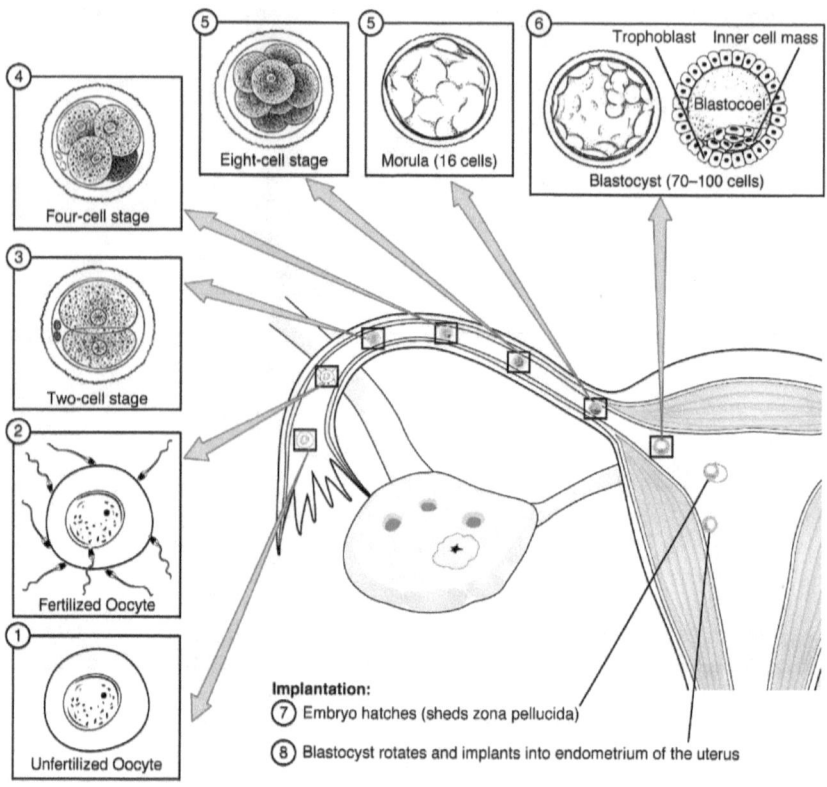

Figure 28.2.2[2] **— Pre-Embryonic Development:** Ovulation, fertilization, pre-embryonic development, and implantation occur at specific locations within the female reproductive system in a time span of approximately 1 week (Biga et al. 28.2)

In IVF, the process of fertilisation is the same; only this happens outside the body. For a viable embryo to form and get to the implantation stage, normal cell division must occur. Embryos are

---

[2] *Images, from Anatomy & Physiology by OpenStax, are licensed under CC BY except where otherwise noted. CC BY 4.0 Deed | Attribution 4.0 International | Creative Commons*

transferred into the womb on Day 2–3 or Day 5–6 as was later explained to me by the doctors. According to the explanation in the diagrams, this can be viewed as either a morula at its 16-cell stage of development (also known as the cleavage stage) or a blastocyst before it reaches the embryonic stage and implants into the uterine wall. Whether this knowledge answers any ethical questions or gives peace to anyone considering IVF treatment is a personal choice.

Arbo is one writer who seeks to answer some of these questions. He discusses the biblical, moral, and ethical aspects of the procedure, and his suggestion is that couples should only have one egg fertilised at a time to avoid creating an excess number of embryos. Indeed, this is an option that some may consider, but it may prove to be an expensive process as the remaining eggs will still need to be frozen for a fee. Doctors may also feel that to fertilise only one egg will not give a good chance of success for someone already having issues conceiving naturally. Certainly, couples can choose to fertilise a small number of eggs at a time if their finances allow it. Maybe, with technology advancing all the time, someday, doctors will be able to pinpoint and retrieve the one egg that will give the highest chance of success. On the other hand, in male infertility, where the sperm may be of poor quality, a procedure called intracytoplasmic sperm injection (ICSI) is used to select the one best quality sperm to inject directly into the egg to maximise the chance of fertilization ("Intracytoplasmic").

We discussed these issues and searched our souls about the decision we were making. Most of all, we sought what God said about IVF. There is no clear reference in the Bible to go by, so we found this question hard to answer. Nonetheless, barrenness in the Bible always preceded a miracle or significant birth which can be traced through to the birth of Jesus Christ. We see this with Sarah and the birth of Isaac (Gen. 21:1-4) who became the father of Jacob. Jacob himself was born after Rebekah his mother had suffered a period of barrenness (Gen. 25:21). From Jacob came the twelve tribes of Israel (Gen. 46:8-27). Rachel gave birth to Joseph, who became governor of Egypt (Gen. 41:37-46). Samuel, who was born to Hannah served as a priest, Israel's last judge and first prophet (1 Sam. 2:18; 7:6, 15-17; 3:20; Acts 3:24). He was to later anoint Israel's King David of the tribe of Judah (Jesus Christ's lineage) (Matt. 1:1-17). Both Sarah and Rachel used concubines or maidservants to bear them children before God opened their wombs. In a way, this was assisted conception, as the concubines acted as what are known as surrogates in today's world. The only difference being that there was physical contact involved in those days whereas today's surrogate does not have physical contact with the male partner.

This still does not offer a tangible answer. There are certainly stories of couples who began their IVF journey and ended up falling pregnant naturally instead or have given birth through IVF only to naturally conceive later pregnancies. This shows that sometimes conception is indeed down to God's timing. For a couple longing for a child or wanting to crack on with making a family, waiting may not seem a wise idea, as it takes a lot of faith to trust God about His timing.

IVF was an option available to us at that time unless God performed a miracle and regenerated my fallopian tubes to enable a natural conception. We still believed this could happen. "For with God, nothing will be impossible" (Luke 1:37). God knew our hearts' desire was to complete our family. We would partner with God so the process would be smooth and not ladened with difficult decisions. Our prayer to God was that the treatment would produce the exact number of embryos for the number of children for which we asked: twins. In Mark 11:24, Jesus encourages us to pray believing in our heart that we have those things that we have asked for and we will receive them.

CHAPTER V

*But if the spirit of Him who raised Jesus from the dead
dwells in you,
He who raised Christ from the dead will also give life to
your mortal bodies through His Spirit who dwells in you.*
— Romans 8:11

For we walk by faith, not by sight.
— 2 Corinthians 5:7

WHEN WE SAW OUR GP, he referred us to a local hospital for fertility investigations, which would be followed by a referral to an IVF clinic. These investigations are for both the man and the woman. They are important as they give a baseline history of the state of both parties' reproductive health. The hope is that any issues with the reproductive system will be picked up and acted upon. A series of blood tests are carried out, which include hormonal tests and a check for sexually transmitted infections.

A semen analysis is performed for the man. This test assesses sperm morphology (the size and shape of sperm), amongst other things. This is important to check, as abnormal sperm can make it more difficult to fertilize the woman's egg. Although it has been established that male infertility affects 7% of the male population, "it is not as often discussed as female infertility partly due to the social and cultural taboos surrounding it" (Latham). The reluctance of some men to get tests done means that some couples spend many childless years focusing on the woman as the one with the fertility issue. This is especially true in Black communities as it can be socially unacceptable for some men to discuss these issues openly or to acknowledge their infertility.

My own tests included a pelvic scan to check the womb. It was during this scan that I first discovered I had fibroids in my womb. On "Overview: Fibroids", the NHS describes fibroids as non-cancerous growths that develop in or around a woman's womb. Women who have fibroids often experience, amongst other things, painful periods, heavy menstrual bleeding, constipation, backaches and passing urine frequently. Statistics show that women from ethnic minority backgrounds, especially those of African-Caribbean origin, are three times more likely to experience fibroids than other ethnicities. The NHS confirms that in rare cases, fibroids can affect pregnancy or cause infertility.

As the specialist IVF doctor that we had been referred to mentioned about my fibroids, I realised I had been living with the symptoms for a long time but never had any proper investigations done. I tolerated my symptoms for years and took them as a part of being a woman. The doctor said the fibroids were outside of the womb and would not affect the implantation of any embryos transferred. She concluded there was no need for any further investigations, though there are other tests that can be done to assess fibroids more clearly, like a hysteroscopy or an MRI scan.

The doctor also made it clear to us that at 40 years of age, I was presenting late for treatment. This took us by surprise because that hadn't crossed our minds. It seems we had not done any research before seeking treatment. The doctor told us that at my age, my ovarian reserve was expected to be low, and my egg quality would likely be poor. This would have a negative impact on our chance of a successful pregnancy. All this new information made us realise how naïve we were in thinking this would be a straightforward process.

She went on to explain that ovarian reserve refers to the number of eggs a woman is estimated to have according to her age. Women are said to be born with all the eggs they will have in their lifetime, and these are released per menstrual cycle. I would later discover that ovarian reserve is measured by a test called Anti-Müllerian hormone (AMH). The AMH varies with age and is at higher levels in younger women if no physiological conditions exist to affect ovarian reserve. The doctor did not check my AMH as part of the investigations, and as we didn't know anything about it then, we did not think to ask why.

Egg quality is another factor that plays an important role in a woman's fertility. Again, scientific evidence shows that the eggs get older as the woman ages, and this contributes to the likelihood of abnormalities like extra or missing chromosomes in the embryo. Chromosomal abnormalities include Down's Syndrome. The doctor said that as I was expected to have poor egg quality, it would have an impact on the fertilisation process and the quality of any embryos produced, which may not implant in the womb lining. Poor egg quality is also linked to miscarriages (Flemming). There was no test to determine egg quality at the time.

During this discussion, I found myself thinking back to when my fallopian tubes were removed when I was younger. Maybe, if I had been in a country with facilities, I would have been advised to freeze my eggs. Medical egg freezing is a procedure that has helped many people realise their dream of being parents if they had to undergo treatment that would affect their fertility, such as chemotherapy. Men can also have sperm frozen medically in such circumstances. Nowadays, egg freezing has become popular in society as more women opt to have children later in life or for the simple reason of not having found the right person to start a family with earlier in life.

After making us understand how low our chance of success was if we were to use my own eggs, the doctor recommended that we use donated eggs from a younger woman instead. She even went as far as to ask if we had considered adoption. We hadn't even thought that far ahead as our naivety had us believing that we would have pregnancy success at the first cycle with my eggs. The thought of using donor eggs was also a surprise, as we weren't aware of such possibilities at the time. What surprised me most was that she would bring up adoption before we had even had one cycle of IVF. We didn't prod as we figured it must be a protocol for doctors to discuss all options for starting a family in the initial stages. However, we informed her that we wished to try with my eggs as we wanted our own biological child.

The surprises did not stop there. All along, we thought the NHS would fund the IVF treatment. We clearly hadn't done enough research, as we were told this would not be the case. The NHS funding for IVF depends on the policy of the local Integrated Care Board (ICB), formally known as Clinical Commissioning Groups (CCGs) or health authority as outlined by NICE. The NHS has given guidance for funding criteria, but the ultimate decision depends on the ICB. At the time, we could not be funded in my then-CCG because of my age and the fact that I already had a child from another relationship. The fact that the child was a young adult, and my husband did not have any children did not change anything.

Despite everything discussed, we did not feel intimidated enough not to go ahead with the treatment. We had no choice as we wanted children, and IVF would make this a possibility. The doctor informed us that she could book us for treatment at her private clinic if we could afford the cost. We went away to consider what our next step would be. We hadn't even set aside any money at that stage.

During that time, we also considered relocating to another part of the country where we could be nearer to family. It made sense to relocate before starting any commitments to treatment. We relocated and took some of the test results with us to show to the next doctor.

Once we'd relocated and felt settled in our new county, we consulted our GP and asked for another referral. We were referred to the local NHS hospital, where investigations would be repeated, only this time, it included a blood test for the AMH. Investigations would be NHS-funded, which we later discovered was a great blessing as the tests cost a lot of money when done in a private practice. We would, however, fund the treatment ourselves, as the protocol for funding was the same as the county from which we had relocated. This time, we were better prepared. We knew which tests would be performed, and we had done research on the cost of IVF. We were keen to start as we were once again reminded that my biological clock was ticking. The hospital was not equipped to perform IVF treatments, but after completing investigations, those eligible for funding would be referred to the affiliated IVF clinic. We had the freedom to choose where we wanted to go as we would be self-funding.

After doing the pelvic scan and seeing the fibroids, the doctor at the clinic referred me for a hysteroscopy at another NHS Trust.

A hysteroscopy is a procedure that looks at the inside of the womb to give a clearer picture than a pelvic scan. I was placed on the NHS waiting list, which could take up to 18 weeks. It was now 2017, and I had turned 41 years old.

Time seemed to be running out. While we were waiting for the hysteroscopy, we started the search for a clinic. There are many private and NHS IVF clinics, and for couples that are self-funding, the choice is endless. People choose a clinic based on various factors like geographical area, prices, reviews, success rates or having been referred by a satisfied customer. Other people prefer to go abroad as prices are more affordable in other countries than in the UK.

As we were searching for a clinic online, the disparities in ethnic representation were apparent in the promotional material provided by most clinics. Compared to the number of Caucasian couples showcased, there were very few clinics showing pictures of couples from ethnic minority backgrounds holding bouncing babies. That was then. Maybe clinics have changed since to show more inclusivity. For a moment, we felt as if we were stepping into a foreign land. This was not surprising as statistics at the time showed that: "IVF was most used by White patients (77%), followed by Asian (15%), Black (3%), Other (4%) and Mixed (2%) patients." IVF Birth rates were lowest in Black and Asian patients; multiple birth rates which contribute to maternal mortality risk were higher in Black patients and Black patients generally started IVF at later ages than other ethnic groups ("Ethnic Diversity").

According to Osei, the delay in seeking fertility treatment by Black people is attributed to several factors such as religious beliefs, isolation, long-held beliefs, and cultural stigma amongst others. Reading these unfavourable outcomes about Black people and fertility treatment sent off alarm bells that we did not want at that point.

It seemed as if the statistics were against us and screaming for us to STOP! Medical statistics are so often deciders of the path doctors take in their patients' medical management and the prognosis they give. Whether they are formal or grapevine accounts, statistics have the potential to either discourage and cast doubt or give hope. Nonetheless, people should know what they are facing whenever they are given a diagnosis. Doctors don't always get it right, but what they don't want is to give false hope. At this point, all we had was our faith. Everything was pointing against us, and none of the doctors who had dealt with us thus far had been optimistic.

It was time to open my own book of statistics. I remembered the women of the Bible whom God had given children in their mature years. Sarah gave birth to Isaac (Gen. 21:2), and Elizabeth gave birth to John the Baptist (Luke 1:5-25). The Bible also says that Isaac prayed for Rebekah, his wife, because she was barren, and God heard his prayer, and she conceived (Gen. 25:21). My husband prayed for me, and God would answer his prayer. Our Christian faith strengthened us into believing that if God had done it before, He would do it again, not for us but for His glory to shine through us. We read our Bible scriptures and declared them over our situation.

God had given life to my mortal body (Rom. 8:11), and that included my reproductive system. He would renew my youth (Ps. 103: 1-5). I believed that God would preserve my youth and make it possible for me to conceive with the use of my own eggs. We acknowledged what the medical statistics said, but we also knew what the ever-living Word of God in our Bible said about faith.

Little did I know that I had entered one of women's most dreaded war zones. There are many war zones in which women find themselves through no choice of their own, war zones such as a relationship breaking down due to broken promises and trust or children suddenly taking a turn and forgetting everything you've ever taught them. Whatever war zone women find themselves in, a strong, positive mindset is key. A conviction that one will emerge the winner, whatever the case may be, is vital, but that's not to underestimate the intensity of some of life's difficult situations that women may find themselves in.

The Bibles says, "Do you not know that those who run in a race all run, but one receives the prize? Run in such a way that you may obtain it" (1 Cor. 9:24). I had to be the one to receive the prize. To achieve that, I needed to arm myself with all the necessary weapons for the battle. One of my weapons was to remain spiritually strong. It was important that I stay connected in church, listening to inspiring sermons and meditating on the word of God in my Bible every day.

CHAPTER VI

*Your wife shall be like a fruitful vine in the very heart of
your house,
Your children like olive plants
All around your table.
Behold thus shall the man be blessed Who
fears the LORD.*
— **Psalm 128:3-4**

As MY HUSBAND AND I PREPARED for the next leg of our journey, I prepared myself for battle as a woman. I continued to meditate daily on the word of God and had a list of scriptures relevant to motherhood pinned onto my wall. As part of our prayer routine, we hung a little girl's dress and a pair of blue mittens on the outside of our wardrobe so we could look at them every day and remind ourselves of what we believed in God for: twins, a boy, and a girl.

We named them and included them in our conversations by name. This might sound ridiculous to some people, but seeing is believing, and faith is calling those things that do not exist as though they did (Rom. 4:17). We had to speak our children into existence.

I prepared myself physically through regular exercise and a healthy diet. A healthy diet is paramount in supporting the body towards a healthy pregnancy and a healthy baby. This healthy practice also extends to the male partner, as sperm production and quality can be affected by poor health habits. In the book of Judges, an angel appeared to Manoah's barren wife to inform her that she was to conceive and bear a son. That son was Samson, one of the strongest men to live, and God used him to judge over Israel and defeat the Philistines. Before he was conceived, the angel gave Manoah's wife specific instructions about her diet:

Indeed now, you are barren and have borne no children, but you shall conceive and bear a son; now therefore please be careful not to drink wine or similar drink, and not to eat anything unclean (Judg. 13:3-4).

This was because Samson was going to be a Nazarite (separated from others and consecrated to God). In today's world, this foundation of healthy living is still relevant for women thinking of getting pregnant.

I also prepared myself psychologically by reducing stress and removing all distracting things from my life. My husband and I needed to create an intimate space to hear from God during this process. I reduced my social media contacts to family and close friends only. I cleared my Facebook account and lost a lot of 'friends' in the process. I looked at fertility blogs and read other women's stories, but I did not let their experiences deter me. When going through medical intervention, it's easy for people to fall into the trap of comparing themselves with other people's experiences. Some experiences are not so favourable, and that can have a negative effect on one's mind before they undergo treatment. I was unique. "Fearfully and wonderfully made" (Ps. 139:14). I was running my own race and staying in my lane.

As we started the journey, we contemplated with whom to share what we were going through. The journey of assisted conception is an intimate one, just as intimate as when people have babies naturally, in my opinion. How many people to tell remains a personal choice, depending on how much support a couple feels they need. Maintaining this privacy can be hard as sometimes, once people are married, the question about when the children will come might pop up, and couples may then be forced to give information away. Sometimes, people are genuinely concerned and come from a place of love, but sometimes, it can be too intrusive. The challenge most women mentioned in their blogs was going back to report the results if things didn't work out. That alone can be emotionally taxing to an already disappointed couple.

From the start, we decided that we would let as few people know as possible as we wanted to avoid having to explain ourselves every step of the way. I told my mum, who already knew my obstetric history. I did not have a live conversation with my mother-in-law about it as I was not ready to tackle this sensitive subject with her. Besides, I was convinced that we were going to be successful and give her a surprise in a few months. We informed some people with whom we were close and considered members of our 'strong army' to pray with us. There is power in agreement in prayer as Jesus promised that if two agree on earth concerning anything that they ask, it will be done for them by the Father in heaven (Matt. 18:19). I did not inform my employer. I didn't want other staff members to get wind of the fact that I was having IVF treatment. I still don't know whether this would have made my journey easier to cope with at work or not. I knew I would need time off for check-ups, but I decided that I would work around it when the time came.

We settled for an NHS clinic in London. At that time, our choice of clinic was determined by cost. It had taken us a while to put the money together for the treatment, and we hoped it would be successful the first time. We paid for the IVF cycle, and it was explained that the price for the actual procedure did not include the medication needed. Our initial thought was that the price was reasonable, but that was before we realised just how much the medication would cost. The drug used to stimulate the ovaries was the most expensive.

The hysteroscopy referral still hadn't come through, and we could not wait any longer. We figured that the doctors at our chosen clinic would do their own assessment and investigations of my womb. They did a pelvic scan but did not suggest anything further. The lead consultant for my treatment said that according to their pelvic scan, the fibroids were outside of the womb and would not affect the implantation of the embryos. There was no need for a hysteroscopy. The only positive thing that surprised even him was that my AMH level was high for my age. Other than that, he wasn't promising anything. Yes, we had entered war territory, but retreat was not the answer.

We approached the start of the cycle with our confidence in God's divine intervention, which would make it possible for us to succeed and prove the doctors wrong. We had a positive mindset, but it was still mixed with some naivety. We were excited for what was to come over the next few months. We believed that nothing was impossible with our God, "… Him who is able to do exceedingly abundantly above all that we can ask or think …" (Eph. 3:20).

The treatment protocol had been explained. The doctors would make a choice of protocol according to an assessment of my medical history. I was placed on what is called a 'long protocol' as the process would take about three to four weeks. I would self-inject hormones for a certain number of days to shut down my natural menstrual cycle (known as downregulation). I would then inject another set of medications to stimulate the ovaries to produce multiple eggs. This would be followed by another injection to mature the eggs for collection. After the eggs had been collected, they would be mixed with the sperm in a dish in the laboratory and left to fertilise. The fertilised eggs would be left to continue cell division until either Day 3 or Day 5, depending on how well the embryo formation process went. The embryologist would make the decision as to what day the embryos would be best transferred into the womb.

As a nurse, the idea of injecting myself was not daunting as my job involved teaching others to inject themselves. In fact, being a nurse helped me easily understand all the medical jargon that goes with fertility treatment, even if I had not worked in that area of nursing. This is not as easy for women who are not in the medical field. Some women have needle phobias, but they must still endure the injections as they are a crucial part of the treatment. My heart goes out to them.

Even though all of this was explained in the beginning, nothing had prepared me for the number of trips we would have to make to the clinic for progress scans. If they are on the long protocol, patients must first have pelvic scans to assess if the down-regulation process worked and that they are ready for the ovarian stimulation phase. During the stimulation phase, scans are done several times to check that the ovaries are responding by producing follicles that contain the eggs. The follicles are measured during the scans as they should be of a certain size before being deemed ready for maturation with the trigger injection.

Then, there were the menopausal side effects during downregulation and the abdominal bloating as my ovaries responded to stimulation. Not to mention that I had to complete all this treatment while still working and had to continue as normal as though nothing was happening. I didn't have to ask for a lot of adjustments at work for these appointments as I was doing shift work, and somehow, most of the appointments seemed to fall on days when I was not working.

Balancing work and fertility treatments is a challenge for most couples. There are not a lot of employers that are flexible enough to give time off for scans and everything else that goes with the treatment. Women are forced to take unpaid time off or use their annual leave days to cover appointments. This has been expressed by most couples in different platforms. Recently, some companies, like Kellogg's, have pledged to be more supportive. In 2021 the company announced that they would be giving extra paid leave to any staff member going through fertility treatments ("Kellogg's"). Through all this, I was consoled by the fact that it would be well worth it once we're holding our babies.

As my treatment progressed, the nurse told me that I was having a textbook response. Hallelujah! I was ready for the trigger injection to mature the eggs and have the eggs collected in the expected timeframe. Egg collection is a delicate procedure undertaken in a theatre under sterile conditions. The patient must sign a consent form beforehand as they must be deeply sedated for the eggs to be collected. Deep sedation is necessary in the egg retrieval procedure as the patient needs to be asleep and not feel any pain. Having had surgery in the past and been under general anaesthesia, I did not have any concerns about being medically sedated. I woke up in a daze afterwards to the doctor telling me the great news that he had managed to collect 12 eggs! It was a very good response for my age, he was happy to say. We went home happy and expectant, thanking God for our success this far. Everything was going smoothly.

We prayed and thanked God for the next step, which was the fertilisation of the eggs. This process is the tricky part because no matter how many eggs are collected, rarely will they all fertilise normally or progress to normal cell division. Twelve eggs did not equal 12 embryos. Embryos are also graded according to quality, and only good-quality embryos are selected for transfer into the womb if there is a good number to choose from.

At home, we eagerly awaited the embryologist to let us know the progress of the fertilisation process. They phoned us on the third day to let us know that the decision was to do a Day 3 transfer. We had three good-quality embryos, and the doctor was happy to transfer all three of them to give me the best chance of getting pregnant. We rushed to the hospital, full of excitement. It would be the first day of the rest of our family's life.

My husband held my hand as I lay on the couch waiting for the doctor who would perform the embryo transfer. I had been told to maintain a full bladder for the procedure, which was not very pleasant. The fibroids made it hard for me to hold a full bladder for long. The doctor scanned me to visualise my womb, but my bladder was not full. I could sense her annoyance as she asked me to drink some more, and she would come back after 30 minutes.

I did that, and after a little wait, our three precious embryos were finally transferred in a straightforward procedure. There was no need for sedation for the procedure, so I was awake throughout. My husband was able to sit with me and hold my hand, and we could chat. We went home armed with a pack of progesterone medication to use as pregnancy support. Women need high levels of progesterone after embryo transfers with IVF. Supplementation is necessary as the body cannot produce the high amounts needed by itself. Progesterone is a hormone produced in the ovaries that is responsible for thickening the womb lining, which is necessary to "sustain embryo endometrial implantation and ongoing pregnancy" (Bulleti et al.).

We bought a pregnancy test on our way home as we had been instructed to do a test on Day 12. This period of waiting is popularly known as the two weeks wait as the pregnancy test must be done between 10 and 14 days. This waiting time is one of the most emotionally draining periods for any couple going through IVF. It is during this time that the embryo is supposed to implant itself in the uterine lining and continue growing. It was explained to me that performing a pregnancy test too early will give false results as the medication used to trigger the maturation of the eggs may still be in the bloodstream. I had three embryos in me, and we were confident that twins were possible. I was also advised that there was no need to take time off work or spend time in bed, so I went back to work to keep my mind occupied. We prayed and thanked God for the lives He was creating. I cannot say what I felt in my spirit, but I had faith in God that He had taken us this far and He would see us all the way.

On the twelfth day, we woke up excited and apprehensive at the same time. We did the test. Negative. We only had one, so my husband went to buy another one, and we repeated the test. Again, a clear negative.

What did I feel? I was numb with disappointment. I did not believe the test, but I knew deep down my heart that it was true, though I wanted it to be an error. I cried helpless tears, knowing we could not change anything. The doctors had been right after all. My eggs weren't good enough. My husband tried as best he could to comfort me.

We phoned the clinic and were told that I should come off the progesterone medication. The turn of events was a bitter pill to swallow. We were empty-handed after spending thousands of pounds and investing ourselves emotionally. It was hard. Despite what the doctors had said about our chance of conception being low, this had taken us by surprise. By faith, we were so convinced I would be pregnant by that time. We hadn't even prepared ourselves for the eventuality that the treatment would not work.

The Bible says, "Now faith is the substance of things hoped for, the evidence of things not seen" (Heb. 11:1). Had we not exercised our faith properly? Surely, we had believed in God. We would like to believe that we obeyed God's word. We trusted what the word of God says in the Bible. We prayed according to that word. We combated doubt by speaking words of faith. We acted and brought ourselves to this place to allow God to work on our behalf. So, what did we not do right?

The failure of an IVF cycle is a tragic time for any couple. Hopes are dashed. Faith is tried. Answerless questions are asked. Relationships are challenged. Preparations made in faith and hope become a painful reminder to be locked away for another time. Finances dwindle, and the question of further funding comes to mind. No couple wants to keep paying the exorbitant price of IVF treatment, but for most, the desire to have children means that money ceases to be an issue. It's a time of emotions: anxiety, stress, depression, anger, sorrow, shame, and rejection. All these feelings are expressed by women in some of their blogs. I felt a deep sorrow and emptiness. I felt guilty as it was my body's failure, and there was nothing wrong with my husband's seed.

My husband continued to comfort me in the coming days, but I was aware that I needed to comfort him, too. This was his loss, too, but I just didn't know how. After all, I felt as if I had failed him. I tried hard to create a normal environment for us by not crying all the time in his presence, but sometimes, I needed that vulnerability because a hug was comforting. Sometimes, I would just curl up in a ball and try to bury what had happened. It wasn't possible to just forget in a hurry.

Couples have different ways of coping at these times. Some people mention going for therapy. Most clinics offer counselling at any stage of the treatment, but we did not take up this offer. Somehow, we felt as if we would not benefit from a cultural, spiritual and ethnicity point of view. Frankly, I was not in the mood to open to anyone. Those who have taken the counselling highly recommend it. Some people take various forms of meditation, join a support group, or engage in vigorous exercise. Whatever works for an individual is usually worth doing because locking oneself up in grief and isolation does not help.

Our help comes from the Lord (Ps. 121:2), so we looked to the heavens and thanked God for bringing us to this stage because we had learnt a lot along the way. I had to pick myself up and go back to work and carry on as though nothing had happened. I told my mum, and she comforted me as a mother would.

At the review appointment, the doctor explained that the failure was probably due to poor egg quality because of my age. He also had another idea: to examine my womb properly to make sure that the fibroids weren't hindering implantation. He then recommended that I have a hysteroscopy before trying for another cycle. I wished he had done this before the first cycle, but looking back was not the answer. We had to think about what was next. In the meantime, we comforted ourselves in the knowledge that God had all the answers. There was a reason why it hadn't happened this time.

CHAPTER VII

It is the Spirit who gives life; the flesh profits nothing.
The words that I speak to you are spirit, and they are life.
—John 6:63

LIFE GOES ON. When we had recovered emotionally, we decided that it was time to try again as we were racing against time. Our idea was to go back to the same clinic and continue with the doctor's recommendation to have a hysteroscopy. The original NHS referral for the test had come through when I was in the middle of the IVF cycle, and I could not have it done then. We could not go back on the NHS waiting list as that would take more time. The doctor referred us to his colleague at a private clinic, and we were given a quotation. The procedure would cost a fair bit. We had a certain amount of money in hand at the time, and we calculated every penny.

It was as we were getting ready to pay for the hysteroscopy procedure that we came across an NHS clinic offering a three-cycle package with the cost of drugs included. We made our calculations and realised that we could pay for the package with the money we had rather than channel it into the hysteroscopy and only one cycle. Even though we had not lost hope, we were now open to the possibility that we might need more cycles before experiencing a successful pregnancy. A three-cycle package would give us peace of mind, and if we were successful the first time, the clinic would give us a refund. We informed the current clinic of our decision and requested that our notes be transferred to the package clinic. We knew the hysteroscopy was still pending, but we trusted that the doctors at the next clinic would take care of it. I was 43 by then, and time was ticking fast.

At the consultation, we first met with the embryologist. We listened as he talked about our chance of success, which sounded too good to be true. We were beginning to wonder why the previous doctors hadn't been as optimistic. It was only after he asked how old I was that his tune changed. He immediately told us to forget everything he had said as he hadn't noted my age. In view of my age, he went on to say, our chances were very low, and their clinic policy didn't allow for women to have treatments with their own eggs after the age of 44. I'm sure he learnt a lesson about consulting patients before confirming the biological data first.

The next appointment was with the doctor. We had done our tests before the consultation, so she was aware of the fibroids. We mentioned that I had been due a hysteroscopy, and we were still keen to have one. She informed us that their pelvic scan had shown that the fibroids were outside of the womb, and their team did not think it was necessary to remove them as it would risk injuring the womb. I asked if it would be possible to freeze any embryos produced from the pending cycle and have the fibroids taken out before they were transferred into my womb. My husband and I had discussed this beforehand, and we were aware of the potential risk of injuring the womb during surgery, but we were willing to take that risk and put everything in God's hands. The doctor said this would not be necessary, and they were happy to proceed. She pointed out that the only issue that might cause it to fail was my egg quality. If I am to be honest, I found the doctor flippant in her approach, and I couldn't shake the feeling that her attitude said, 'Why bother?' Our hands were tied; we were already there, and time was not on my side. We had used up all our money as well, so we had no other options.

One thing that stood out for me at that point was that this was the fourth doctor to assess the fibroids, but they all had a different approach. It became clear to me that there was no set protocol when it came to proceeding with women who presented for fertility treatments with fibroids. All the clinics we had attended were NHS clinics — surely, there had to be a set standard. In my heart, I knew I wanted the fibroids to be taken out, but we had to trust the doctors' expertise.

The treatment commenced, and once again, I was placed on the long protocol cycle. I was familiar with the process and the side effects, so I was, therefore, able to manage. I continued to optimise my health, and so did my husband. When the first cycle failed, I knew it was time to put more effort into my physical well-being. Particularly for women, there are many 'wise people' on the Internet who advise what to eat and drink to improve the chance of IVF success. There are a lot of tailored diets and exercise routines that promise to improve egg quality and improve the womb lining. Some women also share what worked for them. The decision to follow this advice is a personal one, but most women going through fertility treatments are willing to try anything that might give them even a potential ray of success. I tried some licenced products, but I was careful not to compromise my health in the process. I learned that the womb lining is a contributing factor to the successful implantation of the embryo, and the thicker it is, the better. I came across some medical information that stated that there was no product on the market that could improve egg quality. Even though I was taking these products, I also relied on my spiritual faith and trust in the word of God, particularly the Bible verse Romans 8:11. I increased my water intake as this helps with the menopausal side effects of the treatment.

I felt stronger during this cycle, and it was soon egg collection day. On that day, the doctor came to speak to me and gave me the consent forms to sign. I will never forget the words she said to me: "We will go in and collect as many eggs as we can get, but don't expect 12 eggs this time." I felt like a naughty child who had done something they shouldn't have. I did not ask her what she meant, but I figured that she was telling me that I had grown older and to expect 12 eggs was a dream. I woke up later to her telling me that she had collected five eggs. What I don't remember her mentioning was that she had collected eggs from only one ovary, as I was still sleepy. We got only one embryo from that cycle, which was transferred on Day 3. I bled before completing the two-week waiting period.

It was time to cry again and for my husband to comfort me. I know that in his private moments, my husband was drawing strength from God. A lot of emphasis is placed on the woman during IVF treatment, as many couples will testify. Some men have mentioned how medical staff almost always address the woman during consultation and treatment procedures. When cycles fail, more care is given to the woman, but men also experience the loss. Counselling offered by clinics includes the man, but outside of that, there are few support systems tailored to men compared to those supporting women. It is even more difficult in Black and other ethnic minority communities as, culturally, it is not as common for men to discuss such issues openly.

Our only comfort at the time was that we had at least two other cycles already paid for.

After a while, we recovered and prepared ourselves for the next cycle. We continued engaging in life's normal activities, which included work, family, church worship and volunteering services.

It was important for both of us to continue living normal lives and not let IVF take over everything. I continued my health and fitness regime and thinking positive thoughts. Different women have different ways of coping in between cycles, but the most important thing is to stay away from anything that might have a negative psychological impact. I liked reading the testimonies of women in their forties who've had successful pregnancies. There aren't many, but they are there.

COVID-19 hit the country before our next cycle. It meant we had to wait for the clinic to arrange a new way of running programmes. It also meant a small delay, which made me panic as my forty-fourth birthday was fast approaching. I was also expected to self-isolate for the period I would be on treatment as my cycle would be cancelled if I tested positive for COVID. I was eventually booked in and placed on the long protocol again. During this cycle, my follow-up pelvic scans were even more challenging. The right ovary had always been difficult to visualise and was documented as being too high. The scanning nurses continued to struggle to visualise it until the advanced stage of stimulation when there were more eggs (follicles). I am sure this was conveyed to the doctors, as I was told that meetings were held in the afternoons to discuss patients.

The side effects were harder to bear this time, and the nurse said that my body was working very hard on the inside. I felt very tired towards the end. The embryologist suggested we use ICSI as a method of fertilisation this time. ICSI has an added cost and is not routinely recommended, but it is a method of fertilisation in special circumstances. I cannot clearly remember why the embryologist recommended it, but we were prepared to do anything the professionals deemed safe to maximise our chances at that point.

On egg collection day, I had a different doctor than the last time. She sounded more optimistic. I had responded well to treatment, and she told me they were expecting a lot of eggs. I thanked God for He was still holding my hand, and He would not leave me. My husband could not come in with me due to COVID-19 restrictions at the time. I woke up in the recovery area later, and the doctor told me the best news ever: she had collected 14 eggs! It had been difficult to access my right ovary, and the procedure had taken longer than expected. She had worked hard as she knew I had a lot of eggs in my right ovary. I thanked her, and we remembered her in our prayers as she was like an angel God had sent in our time of need.

She was so concerned for my safety that she called me the following day to check if I was all right, as my right ovary had been so difficult to get to. I was well and did not feel any different than the other times after egg collection. I had the usual mild pain and bloating, but it was all worth it as we felt this was the cycle we had been waiting for. Maybe the adrenalin of having sensed a ray of hope was taking away all the pain. During the days that followed, the embryologist gave us some more good news: two of our embryos had done very well, and they were going to be cultured to the blastocyst stage (Day 5). God had been faithful.

Could these be the twins we were hopeful for? We were so happy. We felt that we had finally arrived.

Again, on embryo transfer day, my husband could not go in with me because of the pandemic restrictions. There was no one to hold my hand, but I knew that God was with me. I panicked when I saw a new doctor waiting to perform my embryo transfer. She told me that she would be doing the procedure under supervision. I remember thinking that I should question it as there were concerns about my womb due to the fibroids. What I wanted was for the doctor who had collected the eggs and knew my anatomy to perform the transfer, but I didn't say anything. As a healthcare professional myself, I didn't want to come across as being difficult for my colleagues. The plan was to transfer both embryos. I asked how safe it would be if I fell pregnant with twins in a uterus with fibroids. The embryologist said another set of words that would stay with me forever: "Twins are highly unlikely at your age, and the aim here is to get you pregnant, never mind twins." I felt stupid. She could have chosen kinder words and a gentler tone to convey what she knew to be the truth based on her expert knowledge. I wasn't in denial; I was just a hopeful patient.

At that moment, I was merely thinking about saving our other embryo for another time because my inner self was telling me that things were not right that day, but it was probably too late to request that they freeze one. I closed my eyes and prayed under my breath as the less experienced doctor began the procedure. She was looking at the monitor, and I remember her saying that she couldn't see properly, to which my experienced doctor told her to push the catheter with the embryos in it anyway. Those words still haunt me today. It dawned on me then that to them, I was one of a thousand patients they attended to, and their job was to complete the transfer and move on to the next. They didn't stop to consider that this was my special moment. Those two embryos represented hours of prayer and belief. They represented thousands of pounds spent. They were our two angels that we had already named, and I needed to go out there and confidently say to my husband that we had done it. Even though the statistics had written me off, I was still there trying, and I needed someone to believe with me, even if they did not feel it.

The doctor implanted the embryos somewhere in my womb. She showed me images on the screen, which didn't really mean anything to me, and reassured me that she had placed the embryos far away from the fibroid. I wondered which one she was talking about, as I had been told I had multiple fibroids. As I got off the couch, I knew deep down in my heart that this was a failed transfer. My heart bled as I answered that I was all right when the nurse asked me, and I faked a smile. I knew I should have stopped the procedure and followed my heart. What I wanted was to freeze the embryos and go away to remove the fibroids first. The doctors hadn't suggested this, and I don't know whether they had considered it. Once again, we followed the medical advice. I doubt if I would have been listened to, but I'll never know now. As a healthcare professional, I know that consent can be withdrawn at any time. Patients are permitted to change their minds even at the last minute, but I hadn't heeded my own training.

Once again, I bled before the end of the two-week waiting period. The failure was so hurtful as it was the closest, we had come to conceiving. God had answered our prayers and given us the two perfect embryos. We felt the fibroids in my womb had a lot to do with that failure, yet my doctors still hadn't thought of looking into it. To them, even without the fibroids, my eggs were too old to produce strong embryos.

After that cycle, my confidence was shaken. It is at times like this, when we are down, that the enemy visits to give us one last kick. It is at times like this that he starts to plant seeds of doubt. What if the next cycle didn't work? What if God never intended for us to have children together? These questions came to my mind, but I did not voice them. Voicing them would be like willing them into existence. "Death and life are in the power of the tongue and those who love it will eat its fruit" (Prov.18:21). This was not the time to speak death into what we knew to be God's plans for us: to be a complete family with our biological children. The Bible reminds us "Delight yourself also in the Lord and He shall give you the desires of your heart" (Ps. 37:4). I had to hold on to that promise.

The next cycle would be the last in the package. After we had recovered psychologically and emotionally, my husband and I decided to take control of the situation and have the fibroids reassessed before the next cycle. We didn't want to have another cycle with the fibroids in my womb. My pelvic area was getting more uncomfortable, and we were convinced that the fibroids — and not poor egg quality — made it difficult for the embryos to implant. I responded well to treatment, and my ovaries produced a high number of eggs compared to other women my age. I knew this from reading stories written by other women online. Surely, there was one good-quality egg or more waiting. At our own initiative, we requested my scans from the clinic, which showed the dimensions and positions of the fibroids; I was ready to have them removed.

We searched online for a fibroid specialist. After going through some profiles, we settled on one of the best in London, according to the reviews. We couldn't go through the NHS as the pandemic had increased NHS referral waiting lists, and it could be months before I was seen. The private consultation fee wasn't cheap, and the potential fees for the surgery weren't going to be cheap, but when you want a baby and you have already spent thousands of pounds in currency, another pound extra doesn't matter. We had stopped counting the pounds a long time ago. God was faithful and kept providing the financial means for us to keep paying: "And my God shall supply all your needs according to His riches in glory by Christ Jesus" (Phil. 4:19).

We made contact, and the doctor consulted us through a Zoom video call as it was during the pandemic. The doctor assessed my fibroids through the scans we had sent him from the IVF clinic. He asked questions relevant to women suffering from fibroids. He went by what was in front of him and the measurements presented from the clinic scans. His assessment was that the fibroids were too small to be removed. There was the risk of injuring my womb in the process if he tried taking them out, he said. If the clinic said they weren't affecting the womb lining, he didn't feel there was the need to remove them. He advised that I take vitamin D supplements to boost fertility. Once again, we trusted the specialist. I wish he had been diligent enough to do his own investigations. Maybe then he would have had a clearer picture.

We took his report to the IVF clinic, and they booked us in for the last cycle. We always prayed for a supernatural shift so the fibroids would disappear from my womb. This was the moment we needed God to deliver.

VIII

CHAPTER

For as he thinks in his heart, so is he.
— Proverbs 23:7

*Finally, brethren whatever things are true, whatever things are noble,
whatever things are just, whatever things are pure,
whatever things are lovely, whatever things are of good report,
if there is any virtue and if there is anything praiseworthy — meditate on these things. The things which you learned and received and heard and saw in me, these do, and the God of peace will be with you.*
— Phillipians 4:8-9

WE WENT INTO THE FOURTH cycle with the same optimism we always had but also with a bit of apprehension, as this was the last cycle in the package. This time, the doctor scanned me for herself the day before the egg collection as the nurses continuously struggled to visualise my right ovary during stimulation. She didn't locate it because of the fibroids. She could visualise my left ovary well, and it showed a good response. I knew there were eggs in my right ovary as I could feel them. Experience is a good teacher; somehow, she did not cancel the cycle. On the morning of the procedure, she informed me that if she couldn't locate the right ovary, she'd have to abandon the procedure rather than risk injuring the surrounding organs. My last egg retrieval procedure had been difficult enough, and she was inclined to err on the side of caution. My heart sank even though what she was saying made sense.

I prayed hard in my cubicle as I was being prepared for theatre. I asked Jesus to perform one more miracle. Once again, my husband could not hold my hand as he was not allowed in due to COVID-19 restrictions. After the procedure, the doctor came to let me know that she had only managed to retrieve five eggs from my left ovary and had not visualised my right ovary. In my groggy state after the sedation, I felt a sense of defeat come over me. I had given it my best shot, but here I was, back to square one. We drove home in a sombre mood.

The embryologist called in the afternoon to inform us that only one egg had been fertilised, and they were monitoring it. We had paid extra again for the ICSI procedure, and we prayed that Jesus, who had raised Lazarus from the dead, would do it again (John 11:38-44) to give a fighting spirit to our little embryo. It was not to be, as on the third day, the embryologist called to let us know that the embryo had not made it and there would be no embryo transfer procedure this time.

We received the news, and time seemed to stand still. It was the most heart-breaking news of our journey because it spelt the end of the road. We had run out of time, out of cycles and out of money. The crying began, but this time, it was different. It was more heart-wrenching, and it felt as though my breath was being taken away. In the past, I had cried, but I knew there was another chance. Not this time.

I cried and cried like I had never cried before. It's impossible to describe in words what I felt. Only a woman who has been in the same position will understand. In the coming days, there was a black cloud over me that I felt would never ever be lifted. My husband did his best to comfort me. Again, I knew that I should comfort him, but I didn't know how. I felt as if I had failed him and his family. I felt as if I had failed to carry on his legacy in my assignment as a woman. I enveloped myself in my grief and just cried all the time in private. I didn't want my husband to see my tears all the time. I phoned the clinic to ask for a sick note to stay away from work. They advised me to call my GP and offered counselling, but I was beyond counselling. I didn't want to talk to anybody about it.

Phoning the GP seemed too much of a task, so I summoned up the strength and went back to work after a few days of recovery from the pain of the procedure, but my heart ached. I was glad for the face mask as I could not fake a smile at work. I tried hard to carry on as normal, but I cried with my heart at every opportunity when I was alone, biting back the tears so no one would see them; it was a good thing I wore spectacles. I couldn't pray. I didn't know what to pray. I couldn't open my Bible. I just wanted to be left alone. I was having a solo pity party, and I wasn't about to invite anyone. Nothing anybody could have said would have been helpful at that moment. I had questions for God. Why had He not let it happen? What were we missing? What was His plan for our marriage if we couldn't have children? It seemed that the enemy had finally delivered that last kick.

There are, unfortunately, some Christian women reading this who will judge me for not having been more prayerful at the time, but fortunately, there are other Christian women who recognise that a circumstance can present you with a test you haven't prepared for. I hadn't prepared myself for this. I had prepared for a pregnancy. There are some situations in life that knock the sails out of you, and you are left stunned and dumbfounded. The Apostle Paul instructed the Thessalonians to "Rejoice always, pray without ceasing, in everything give thanks …" (1 Thess. 5:16-18). I don't know if he considered a forty-something-year-old woman who had just had her fourth cycle of IVF fail and been told it's the end of the road.

Somehow, in my grief, there was a distant peace, a distant stillness in my heart that I could not explain. Sometimes, I suddenly stopped crying and felt an overwhelming sense of peace come over me. It was a conflicting sense of emotions considering what was happening. I knew then that the peace of God that surpasses all understanding was guarding my heart and my mind (Phil. 4:7), so that even if the enemy had kicked me, I would not fall overboard. I did not forget that God was there; I just could not communicate with Him in my grief-stricken state except to ask questions.

In the coming weeks, as I thought over things in my heart, I realised that the enemy had me where he wanted me. He had driven me to cower in a corner in a state of confusion, a state of loss, a state of shame and a state of worthlessness. He was willing me and pushing me to sink deeper and pulldown what God had put together. I realised then what a thin line there was between making it out of a tragic situation and never being able to come out of it. It was a light bulb moment for me. I was at a crossroads. Either I could turn right and pick myself up and remember who I was in Christ, or I could turn left, sink deeper and end up in a state of depression, probably having to pop a pill a day just to make it to the next.

I was on the brink of ill mental health. Some of life's unpleasant situations have the potential to throw people at a crossroads like this. It doesn't mean that those who turn left are any weaker. Sometimes, it's about the support systems around that person when things happen. I turned right, and I remembered my support system. I visited memory lane and reminded myself how far God had taken me. This was not the first battlefield I had found myself in. I remembered what I had heard some people say in the past; 'This too, shall pass!' The Bible reminds us that:

> *This light, temporary nature of our suffering is producing for us an everlasting weight of glory, far beyond any comparison, because we do not look for things that can be seen but for things that cannot be seen. For the things which are seen are temporary, but the things which are not seen are eternal* (International Standard Version Bible, 2 Cor. 4:17-18).

I had to zoom out and look at the situation from another angle. I had to stop engaging in conversations with the serpent like Eve did (Gen. 3:1-6). I could hear the serpent whisper, 'Did God actually say you will have children'? I needed to replace that with something else to shut it all out. I heard instead the young preacher Jakes Roberts say the words, "Girl, Get Up!"

I got up and I remembered my support system, the living Word of God, in my Bible. God says that I should fear not for He is with me (Isa. 41:10). The book of Psalms says that He will cover me with His feathers and under His wings I will take refuge (Ps. 91:4). No evil shall befall me (Ps. 91:10). I should lift my eyes to the hills for my help comes from Him (Ps. 121:1). I am a fruitful vine in my husband's household and my children are like olive plants around his table (Ps. 128:3). I should delight myself in Him, He will give me the desires of my heart (Ps. 37:4). "I can do all things through Christ who strengthens me" (Phil. 4:13). His Word stands true yesterday, today, and forever more. I read a book at this time by Meyer titled *Battlefield of the Mind* that told me I needed to conquer my mind before the enemy turned it into his playfield.

I reminded myself that I was a mother and a wife first before I was an IVF patient, and my husband needed his wife back. This was not the only issue we were facing in our lives. There were other areas of our lives that needed both of our attention. My husband and I were a part of the pastoral team at the church we attended at the time. Part of our role was to pray for others in the congregation. There were people going through worse situations in life. Some were life-and-death situations. I had to remind myself that I was still alive, and I still had my health. I had to meditate on all things good and believe that the peace of God would be with me (Phil 4:8). It was time to count my blessings and be thankful. There was another woman elsewhere going through the same situation as me, and maybe even worse than me. I had a husband who, despite facing the challenges of not being a father yet amongst his peers, was still there, holding my hand and never once losing hope. My son needed a mother's guidance as he was navigating adult challenges of his own. The wider family circle needed us to connect and be involved in family matters. The journey of infertility and fertility treatment can cause a lot of stress and strain on relationships as couples struggle to balance the emotions that come with it while dealing with everyday life issues.

I travelled down memory lane and remembered how God had been there time and time again in my moments of crisis, always a still small voice and imaginary arm around my shoulders telling me it was going to be all right. He was not about to let go of me now. Life had to go on. I remembered the old saying, 'Don't throw the baby out with the bathwater.' I had to put the gloves back on and enter the ring again. I did not know what God's next move would be, but I was willing to listen. I was curious.

I chinned up, cleaned myself up and got ready to face the world. The tears would still come now and again, but I was ready for God's next step. It would start with a visit to the beach in Kent with my husband on a sunny weekend afternoon. As we sat on that beach, my husband's arms around me, we talked about letting his family know about the state of things. We talked about the next step we didn't have. We had not planned to be there. By rights, we should have been there with our children playing games on the beach.

My anxiety was letting my mother-in-law know that we had reached the end of the road. I had never had an open conversation with her about the infertility. I felt as if I hadn't yet worn my woman's crown in the family, and time was not on my side, but the conversation had to take place. I needn't have worried because my mother-in-law believed in God. She had been praying for us all along, and I was overwhelmed by the amount of support she had given me. She reminded me of her love for me as a daughter and that she loved me as I was. She said that we should trust God as He had a plan. I felt ashamed for not having been more open.

CHAPTER IX

*And to the angel of the church in Philadelphia write these things, says He who is Holy, He who is true, He who has the key of David,
He who opens, and no one shuts and shuts, and no one opens;
'I know your works. See, I have set before you an open door,
and no one can shut it; for you have a little strength, have kept My word and have not denied my name.*
— Revelation 3:7-8

"Go up now, look toward the sea." So, he went up and looked and said, "There is nothing." And seven times he said, "Go again."
— 1 Kings 18:43-46

IN THE WEEKS THAT FOLLOWED, my husband and I prayed, seeking wisdom from God, to hear from Him what we should be doing next. The church we attended at the time had reopened since the pandemic, and I started attending church physically once more. Gradually, I felt the healing in my heart, and I started engaging in normal conversations with people. The ache was still there, especially as several couples seemed to have had babies during the isolation period. A new baby announcement at church or noticing that another couple were pregnant again still brought on that little tug in my heart. I was happy for everyone, but it was hard not to long for the day when we would be announced as the new parents. One day, I listened to a message about the God of time, about how God was never late; He was always on time. I felt that message speaking to me that day. At that moment, God reminded me that He had not said it would not happen. He was just saying not yet, but like Sarah in the Bible, I didn't see how it would happen.

In time, my husband and I sat down to explore our situation again. When couples have failed to conceive through their own gametes (egg and sperm), several options are present. Depending on the medical issue, couples can use donor eggs, donor sperm or donor embryos. The option to use donor eggs had been mentioned during our journey, and we approached this idea with an open mind. Donor parenting has certainly become more popular in recent years, but it just did not sit well with us. Our desire was to have our biological children with both of our DNA. My honest feeling was that I would always have a 'Hagar' moment and feel as if there was a third woman in our marriage.

We came across stories of children born via donor gametes. In one story, one man's relationship with his parents had been destroyed as he felt that his parents had no right to create him when he could not trace his biological parents. His parents had used donor sperm and donor eggs to conceive. On the other hand, one woman felt so loved and grateful that her parents had used a donor egg and had wanted her so much that she had no desire to find her other biological parent ("My shock"). The commonality of donor parenting in our society and some of the complexities that arise from it are highlighted in the documentary *And Me: My Sperm Donor and Me.*

Currently, in the UK, the law allows people born from donor gametes to have identifiable information about their donor parent disclosed when they turn 18 years old if requested. This law is subject to change in the future as proposals are being made for it to be 'amended to enable the removal of donor anonymity from the birth of any child born from donation' ("Modernising"). We discussed navigating the new complexities if the child decided to start a relationship with their other biological parent.

The most important thing for us was God's view on the issue. As I mentioned earlier, in the Bible, the women Sarah, Rachel and Leah are documented to have given their maidservants to their husbands to bear children on their behalf. These are isolated stories highlighted in the Bible, but this may well have been common practice in those days. In a way, they were using donor eggs, only there was actual physical contact. We wanted to listen to God's voice on this, and after praying over the situation, we concluded that donor parenting was not for us, even if there were no options left.

Then there was adoption. We talked about it, but it seemed like closing a door that God hadn't said should be closed. We parked the thought to revisit it later.

Most of all, we asked God to show us His will, so we didn't make any mistakes going forward. Many times in life, we make decisions and ask God to intervene in the decisions we have already made. How do we discern if something is, indeed, God's will or the Holy Spirit leading us to take the steps we are taking? This is explained in a compilation of stories by DeCenso Jr. In this book, contributors share the various ways in which God communicates with us and how we can cultivate our ability to listen. Some of the ways mentioned are: God may send a prophetic word through an anointed person and sometimes through visions and dreams. Other times, it's the inner peace we feel that tells us this is the Holy Spirit leading us. Hearing from God and hearing Him clearly is a delicate process. If we don't, we sometimes end up taking the long route to our destiny by leaning on our own understanding. This is confirmed in the scripture, "Trust in the Lord with all your heart and lean not on your understanding; In all your ways acknowledge Him and He shall direct your paths" (Prov 3:5-6).

My husband suggested that we search for another clinic that would treat me with my own eggs at my age. When he mentioned it, I was still optimistic, but at the same time, I was apprehensive as I did not want to be disappointed. My husband has never been one to give up easily. I agreed in the end because I figured that God was communicating something to him.

Before we restarted the search, I dreamt of myself trying to shut a door, but try as I might to push it, I couldn't because there was a force behind the door, keeping it open. I remember being scared in the dream as it was dark behind the door. All I could feel was a strong force keeping me from shutting it. I woke up to find my husband gently shaking me and telling me I was talking in my sleep. I told him about the dream, and we concluded that maybe it was because I was trying to shut a door that God wanted to remain open.

And God, indeed, opened a door that blew us away. Not far from where we lived, there was a private clinic whose protocol allowed for me to be treated with my own eggs until the age of 46. I had just turned 45 years old at the time. We called a lot of clinics that didn't have this protocol in place at the time, so this was an amazing opportunity for us. The price of treatment at this clinic was very high, but we didn't think of the cost this time. All we needed was to be accepted for treatment. We were so excited as we booked the appointment, as suddenly, there was a ray of hope. We prayed for the team at the clinic to be receptive and for God to open their eyes to my medical needs.

As we entered the clinic, we both felt at peace. The motto of the clinic was one that gave us hope. I was older, but this fact was not once thrown in my face during the consultation. I was treated as a woman coming in to have IVF treatment, not an 'older woman' with poor egg quality.

The consultation process was straightforward, especially as this would be our fifth cycle, and we knew the drill. I was booked in for my first pelvic scan, which would be followed by what they called a saline infusion sonogram (SAS or SIS) scan. This saline scan closely assesses the womb for any issues that might hinder the implantation of the embryo. It is less invasive than the hysteroscopy I was supposed to have in the past. The consultant proceeded to do my pelvic scan first, and after a few minutes, he said the most encouraging words we had heard in a long time! He said, "I don't need to do the saline scan. I have already seen the problem. It's the fibroids."

Time stood still for me for the second time. It was a life-changing moment. We had spent years and thousands of pounds in IVF treatment being attended to by professionals knowledgeable in their field, but it took only a few minutes for one doctor to diagnose the problem. I got up from the couch, full of confidence that we had come to the right place.

After the scan, the consultant made two drawings on a piece of paper. One was of a normal female reproductive system, showing the womb, fallopian tubes, and ovaries as they should be. The other picture was of my reproductive system, as he had seen it on the scan. The shape of my womb had been distorted by the fibroids. It did not make for a conducive environment for a baby to grow. The fibroids had pushed my right ovary high up, displacing it from its normal position. The largest fibroid obscured my right ovary, which is why the last clinic couldn't visualise it properly.

Without saying much, the consultant asked me what the last clinics had been doing all the years they were treating me. I experienced a mix of emotions as I listened to him map out our next steps. I was angry at being let down by the medical professionals we had trusted to take care of me. I was angry that we had lost two good-quality embryos and possibly a lot of viable eggs when they couldn't collect them in the past. I thought of all the pain from the injections, the side effects of the medications and the emotional stress we had suffered, all because none of the doctors had taken the initiative to decide that the fibroids could possibly be the main issue hindering the process of getting me pregnant. I also felt grateful that the last doctor had not prodded further to try to get eggs from my right ovary, as she could have injured me in the process. Sometimes, it helps to look at both sides of the coin.

The consultant told us that there would be no point proceeding with a cycle with the fibroids still in my womb. We left the clinic with a provisional date to have surgery to remove them. My husband and I went home filled with hope that God had finally opened someone's eyes. The surgery wasn't going to be cheap, as I couldn't do it on the NHS due to waiting lists. There are no waiting lists in private practice, and we had spent so much money up to that point that another few extra pounds didn't matter.

It felt as if the fibroids were aligning with what was about to happen because approximately one week after that appointment, I woke up with the most excruciating pain in my womb. I called emergency services and was referred to my GP, who concluded that my womb was contracting to try to expel the fibroids. He advised that I should wait for my booked surgery date. It was time for them to leave my body. Within a month after seeing the consultant, I was back home, recovering after open myomectomy surgery in which six fibroids were removed. As I recovered at home, I started getting excited about what God had in store next.

CHAPTER X

A man's heart plans his way, but the Lord directs his steps.
— **Proverbs 16:9**

GOD'S TIMING IS THE BEST. This is one of the more popular statements you'll hear Christians say to one another when concluding a situation that seems to be taking too long to break through. Why do we sometimes feel as if God has taken too long to answer our prayers? To answer my own question, I think it's because, as humans, we set our hearts' desires and expect God to act as soon as we let Him know what we want, but God does not operate like that. God does not give us what we want when we want it because sometimes, it might not be right for us at the time.

Indeed, most times, God surprises us with things we have not asked for. If God had it in His plan to make it happen, He would, even if we don't ask. So, when we have a desire and ask of Him, we should trust that He has heard us. Also, God does not always say yes. If it's not a part of His plan and purpose for us, He will shut the door. That is why, in our desires, we should trust that He establishes our steps (Prov. 16:9). It also doesn't always happen the way we want it. Sometimes, there are twists and turns we do not anticipate before we get there. Sometimes, there's an area of growth inside us that needs to happen before God entrusts us with the gift.

As I was recuperating at home from my surgery, I realised that we were operating on God's timing. In our desire to complete our family, I had almost forgotten that. I had thrown tantrums every time the cycle failed, but everything had its time. I had been diagnosed with fibroids for four years up to that point. I had been attended to by four very qualified consultants in the past, but it took only a few minutes for my current consultant to make the decision to take them out. When God's timing is right, things suddenly happen.

Was there a degree of medical negligence? Maybe, but I trust God and His timing. There was a special reason why He had not allowed the surgery to happen before. Fibroids increase in size over time. Maybe it would have been unsafe to take them out before then without injuring my womb. Maybe God knew this doctor would be the one with the expertise to do the job well. Whatever it was, only God knows.

I found the time while healing special because, suddenly, I had slowed down. I didn't have to rush to the next shift at work or the next scan or procedure. I was grounded for the next six weeks as my body needed the time to heal.

I had resigned from my previous job before the surgery and was due to start a new job, but I realised that would be impossible. With everything I had been through, I needed more than the six weeks my doctor had given me as time off to fully regenerate. I had been on the go for a long time, and I wanted to concentrate on my physical and mental health wellbeing. I didn't see how I could throw myself into a new, demanding job. I needed a break. Sometimes in life, it's important to recognise when our bodies, minds and spirits need refuelling, or we risk running on empty, and that does not achieve anything. I discussed this with my husband, and we concluded that I should withdraw from my newly offered position.

This was my time to declutter, prioritise and channel my energy to the right places. I had been through the wine press for a while by then, but God was making new wine (Matt 9:17). My priority was to create an intimate space so I could clearly hear God's voice. We had to get it right this time. I remembered decisions we'd made in the past that might have contributed to the turnout of events. Maybe if we had listened more to God's voice, we would have waited longer for the first hysteroscopy procedure we'd missed. Maybe that would have shaped our path differently. Maybe I should have followed God's voice and spoken up about freezing the two blastocysts we'd lost. Whatever the case maybe, I didn't want to be left with any questions this time.

I knew then that God would finish our story. I don't know how, but I somehow felt that this time, the only tears I would have would be tears of joy. I was older, and the statistics hadn't changed, but I felt confident and at peace. During that time, I strongly felt that I should write our story. I didn't know how God would end it yet, but I knew how I wanted it to end, so I started to write this testimony. The quiet space helped me focus and explore my feelings about the journey we had undergone thus far. In my heart, I felt as if I needed to do my bit and join the other women of colour who have shared their stories, having open conversations about fertility issues, and going through treatment. I had to let others know they were not alone and that their story was not the worst story. Mine wasn't the worst, either.

I had to let women of Christian faith know they should not lose hope because God was always in the middle of it all, that it was all right to have feelings of doubt, fear, anxiety, guilt, pain, sorrow, hopelessness and all the feelings I had while going through my journey that did not seem right. Grieving is a process whether one is Christian or not. The only thing that is not right is to stay in that state and forget to look in the mirror of your identity, which is the Word of God in the Bible.

I especially wanted to let women from underrepresented communities know that it's all right to seek medical help for fertility issues, especially while they are still at an age when the NHS will fund their treatment. Also, everyone who seeks medical attention will not wind up on the IVF route. Other issues can be rectified, such as the removal of fibroids, like in my case. I wanted to tell my story so the next Black woman who presented for fertility treatment with fibroids would receive better care than I originally experienced. Hopefully, regulatory bodies will be prompted to review their policies and procedures in places where women receive care.

After six weeks, at the review appointment, the doctor examined me and was satisfied that I had recovered well from the surgery. I thanked him for the care, but he said, "Don't thank me now. Thank me when the baby comes." I remember thinking that only God's divine intervention could have brought such a doctor into our lives. The lack of ethnic representation in the fertility sector has been raised by some. Johnson shares the following sentiments:

> *Being Black in the infertility world means not seeing your story represented in the very communities it's designed to support. It means not being guaranteed to see a doctor that [sic] looks like you and or [sic] will approach your case with racial sensitivity. It's one of the reasons my communities fight so hard for representation because it matters.*

Perhaps it is not surprising that the doctor who finally took control of my case was Black African.

XI

CHAPTER

Behold I will do a new thing,
Now, it shall spring forth; Shall you not know it?
I will even make a road in the wilderness and rivers in
the desert.
— Isaiah 43:19

AFTER A RECOVERY PERIOD OF THREE months, the clinic booked us for what would be our fifth IVF cycle. It was January 2022, post-COVID. We were at peace we had received good care from the team at the clinic. The doctor opted for the 'short protocol' of treatment. This protocol differs from the long one in that it only lasts for a duration of two weeks. The patient starts injecting medication on Day 1 or 2 of the menstrual cycle. Being on the short protocol, coupled with the fact that I had no fibroids in my womb, meant that I experienced the most comfortable cycle I'd had since starting IVF treatment. There was no pressure in my pelvic cavity, especially on my bladder. My life had improved since the fibroids were taken out as all the symptoms with which I had lived had subsided.

Soon, it was egg collection time. I was sedated again, and I woke up to the wonderful news that the doctor had collected ten eggs from both of my ovaries! We opted for ICSI again as we had done in the past and drove home in an excited mood to await the news of the fertilisation rate. The embryologist called us later that day to let us know the most wonderful news: we had achieved a 70% fertilization rate. We thanked God for everything so far and waited for news of an embryo transfer date.

On the third day, the embryologist phoned with more good news. Six of our embryos were doing well, and the decision was to culture them to the blastocyst stage. This meant we would have a Day 5 transfer! Our God, who can do 'exceedingly abundantly above all we can ever ask or think' (Eph 3:20), had done over and above what we imagined. I had not imagined having so many embryos at that time in my life.

Having six embryos was a marvellous achievement. We had asked God for twins. We found ourselves faced with the question: how would I carry six babies? The answer was easy for us. We asked God, and He had supplied in good measure. We made the decision to have two embryos transferred first and freeze the rest to be transferred later. I prepared myself mentally to spend the rest of my life pregnant! History was being made. Women getting pregnant in their fifties were still making news, and I wondered if I would be one of them.

However, on the morning of the embryo transfer, the embryologist called to say that we had been left with two of the strongest embryos they had selected from the five remaining. One of the embryos had stopped growing on its own. They had removed the rest from the culture as their assessment was that they would not be strong enough to survive the freezing and thawing process in the future. We were disappointed by this news, especially due to the fact we had not been given the opportunity to decide for ourselves if we wanted to freeze them anyway. We had to take the experts' medical advice, and we were grateful for the two that were going to be transferred. This is the one thing about IVF treatment: numbers change at every stage. The number of eggs collected and fertilised is rarely equal to the number of embryos in the end.

We were booked for the embryo transfer that afternoon, and we both went in with a spring in our step. We had waited so long for that moment. This time, it felt right. The staff were warm and supportive. My husband was not allowed into the theatre as there were still pandemic restriction measures in place. I felt a wave of emotions come over me as I lay on the couch, and the embryologist showed me a picture of the two blastocysts that would be transferred. Our twins. It was such an amazing feeling.

The procedure was quick and straightforward, and I was awake the whole time. I could not wipe the smile from my face when I met my husband in reception. We hugged and savoured the moment and left the clinic with smiles on our faces. This time, we looked forward to the two-week wait period.

During the wait, I tried to listen to my body for a sign. My body didn't give me any signs, but my mind was at ease. I was curious to know, though, so I asked God for a dream to show me if I was pregnant. There was nothing, and I didn't dream of anything significant. God was not giving anything away.

On the twelfth day, my husband bought a pregnancy test. For some reason, in our excitement, we hadn't got one in advance. I performed a test, but the test strip didn't work. Anxiety can result in your not reading instructions properly. He went out to buy two more, and we did tests on two separate urine samples.

I screamed while still in the bathroom when my test registered a clear positive! I found him holding his test, which had a clear positive, as well! I fell on my knees and praised my God. He had done it for us in His own perfect time.

At that moment, I felt a load lift from my shoulders. It was almost unbelievable. Our lives had been transformed in an instant. This was the first day of the rest of our lives. The pain of the past quickly faded minute by minute.

We picked up the phone to let the clinic know of our news. They congratulated us and booked us for a five-week scan to determine how many babies I was carrying. We were excited but also mindful this was a delicate stage of pregnancy. We had jumped one hurdle, but there was still the hurdle of carrying the pregnancy to term. We had faith in our God that He would not take us this far, only to take us back to where we had come from. We did not tell anyone else at that stage.

We waited for the five-week scan, which seemed to take forever. The pregnancy was progressing well, though I didn't feel any different yet.

Finally, the day came. Another hurdle. This is the one thing that I learnt about fertility treatment: you are always waiting for the next stage and then praying that you make it to the next. There we were, having made it to the next stage, and I was lying on another couch for another scan. This time, we waited for some heartbeats only to be told that the number had gone down again. One of our embryos hadn't made it, but we had one perfect heartbeat beating away at a very fast pace. Our one miracle was about to complete our family.

We held hands as we enjoyed the moment. The years of pain, hurt and tears that had led to this very special moment were fast becoming a distant memory. God had wiped away my tears of disappointment in an instant. The scanning nurse reminded us of this was a delicate stage of pregnancy. She was gentle in warning us that it's not over till you're holding that baby. I closed my eyes and thanked God, and I heard that still small voice again, this time saying, *"I've got you."* I knew then that everything was going to be all right and that we'd be holding our bundle of joy in a few months' time.

XII

CHAPTER

He who has begun a good work in you will complete it until the day of Jesus Christ.
— Philippians 1:6

He has made everything beautiful in its time.
— Ecclesiastes 3:11

He grants the barren woman a home, like a joyful mother of children.
Praise the Lord!
— Psalm 113:9

As my husband and I paid another visit to the beach (with me heavily pregnant) and to the spot where we had sat the previous year, I couldn't help but remember what the prophet Elisha said to the Shunammite woman: "About this time next year you shall embrace a son" (2 Kgs 4:16). I am reminded how, as I cried at the time, a sense of peace seemed to come over me, and I could almost feel an arm around both of our shoulders comforting us. I know now that God had been making that same promise: *'This time next year.'* We went back to the spot that day to thank God for answering our prayers.

We have a precious little girl now, and we'll take her there one day. She arrived in the autumn of 2022. We originally asked God for two, but we are overjoyed with our gift. It all seemed so distant at one time, but now, it hardly seems as if we waited at all. I look back to where we came from. There must have been a reason for us going through that journey, and for me, the journey started all those years ago on the surgical table when I lost my second fallopian tube. I didn't know where the journey would lead then, but I know now that it has strengthened my faith in God. I know that without my faith, I wouldn't be writing this book. I would probably have crumbled and given up a long time ago. We could have easily been intimidated by the medical statistics at the beginning of our journey and given up, but our faith would not let us. When we look at our daughter, we realise what we would have missed out on if we had given up.

My hope is that anyone reading this book will be encouraged with the knowledge that in life, we are always one step away from that breakthrough, opportunity, or open door. Ours came through one special doctor who saw what the other doctors considered to be trivial when it came to realising our dream. This is our testimony, and I hope it will help another couple on their journey. Our story could have ended differently, but God made a way possible. Many couples have been on this journey only to be left empty-handed at the end, so we do not underestimate what a gift it is to have travelled this far and been successful. It doesn't mean that those who end up empty-handed are not prayerful enough; it means that God has a different plan and purpose for us all even though it's hard to understand sometimes. We share our testimony because it might be the one story that someone needs to hear to keep going.

I encourage all my sisters who are still waiting to never forget that you are fearfully and wonderfully made (Ps 139:14). You are perfect, and not carrying a child does not make you any less. To those couples who have gone through the journey and finished with an empty nest, I pray that you find peace and for God to reveal His divine purpose for you. I truly don't know whether this statement would have helped me if things had ended differently for us. I say this because I know that for most women, there is no greater desire than holding their own child.

I am convinced that my journey as a woman was part of the bigger picture of God's purpose for my life. My experience has birthed so many things including being an author of women's books of faith. I now write books to encourage other women to dig deeper within themselves and discover their God-given purpose amid adversity. I would like to agree with Warren when he writes, "The purpose of your life is far greater than your own fulfilment, your peace of mind, or even your happiness" (17).

Finally, to those who know a woman or couple in waiting, please remember to be considerate and kind. And to those who are still waiting or whose journeys didn't end the way you envisioned, I pray that the 'God of all comfort' continues to comfort you in your specific circumstances in the way He uniquely knows how.

The End.

Motherhood Daily Declarations

I am not alone.

"The Lord is my shepherd; I shall not want. He makes me to lie down in green pastures; He leads me beside the still waters. He restores my soul; He leads me in the paths of righteousness For His name's sake. Yea, though I walk through the valley of the shadow of death, I will fear no evil; For You are with me; Your rod and Your staff, they comfort me."

— Psalm 23:1-4

My body is healed.

"But if the Spirit of Him who raised Jesus from the dead dwells in you, He who raised Christ from the dead will also give life to your mortal bodies through His Spirit who dwells in you."

— Romans 8:11

I wait patiently.

"Wait on the Lord; Be of good courage, And He shall strengthen your heart; Wait, I say, on the Lord!"

— **Psalm 27:14**

I have no anxiety.

"Be anxious for nothing, but in everything by prayer and supplication, with thanksgiving, let your requests be made known to God; and the peace of God, which surpasses all understanding, will guard your hearts and minds through Christ Jesus."

— **Philippians 4:6-7**

I am confident in God's promises.

"Being confident of this very thing, that He who has begun a good work in you will complete it until the day of Jesus Christ."

— **Philippians 1:6**

Nothing is impossible with my God.

"Now indeed, Elizabeth your relative has also conceived a son in her old age; and this is now the sixth month for her who was called barren. For with God nothing will be impossible."

— Luke 1:36-37

God will open my womb.

"Then God remembered Rachel, and God listened to her and opened her womb."

— Genesis 30:22

There is an appointed time for me.

"For Sarah conceived and bore Abraham a son in his old age, at the set time of which God had spoken to him."

— Genesis 21:2

I trust God.

"By faith Sarah herself also received strength to conceive seed, and she bore a child when she was past the age, because she judged Him faithful who had promised."

— **Hebrews 11:11**

God will answer my husband's prayer.

"Now Isaac pleaded with the Lord for his wife, because she was barren; and the Lord granted his plea, and Rebekah his wife conceived."

— **Genesis 25:21**

I am fruitful.

"Your wife shall be like a fruitful vine in the very heart of your house, Your children like olive plants around your table."

— **Psalm 128:3**

God hears my prayers.

"Then Eli answered and said, 'Go in peace, and the God of Israel grant your petition which you have asked of Him.'"
— 1 Samuel 1:17

I believe God.

"Therefore, I say to you, whatever things you ask when you pray, believe that you have them, and you will have them."
— Mark 11:24

Jesus is my strength.

"I can do all things through Christ who strengthens me."
— Philippians 4:13

I will not lose hope.

"Rejoicing in hope, patient in tribulation, continuing steadfastly in prayer."
— Romans 12:12

I have a strong will.

"And not only that, but we also glory in tribulations, knowing that tribulation produces perseverance, and perseverance character, and character hope. Now hope does not disappoint, because the love of God has been poured out in our hearts by the Holy Spirit who was given to us."

— Romans 5:3-5

I am fertile.

"You shall be blessed above all peoples; there shall not be a male or female barren among you or among your livestock."

— Deuteronomy 7:14

God answers my prayers.

"May the LORD answer you in the day of trouble; May the name of the God of Jacob defend you. May He send you help from the sanctuary and strengthen you out of Zion; May He remember all your offerings and accept your burnt sacrifice. May He grant you according to your heart's desire and fulfil all your purpose."

— Psalm 20:1-4

My womb is blessed.

"Then God blessed them, and God said to them, 'Be fruitful and multiply; fill the earth and subdue it; have dominion over the fish of the sea, over the birds of the air, and over every living thing that moves on the earth.'"

— Genesis 1:28

I am a mother.

"He grants the barren woman a home like a joyful mother of children. Praise the Lord!"

— Psalm 113:9

My womb is fruitful.

"Behold, children are a heritage from the Lord, the fruit of the womb is a reward."

— Psalm.127:3

All of God's plans for me are good.

"For I know the thoughts that I think toward you, says the Lord, thoughts of peace and not evil, to give you a future and a hope."
— Jeremiah 29:11

God is always with me.

"Have I not commanded you? Be strong and of good courage; do not be afraid, nor be dismayed, for the Lord your God is with you whenever you go."
— Joshua 1:9

About the Author

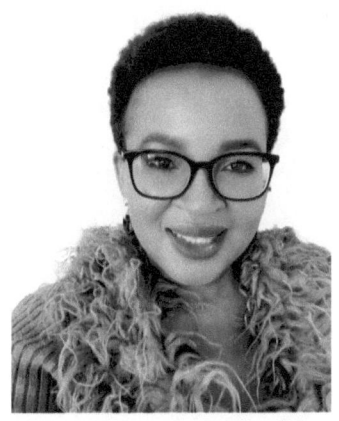

Kwenza Onyenakala is a qualified registered nurse and holds a first-class degree in Sexual Health from the University of Greenwich. She resides in the United Kingdom. Her passion is to use her experience to inspire and encourage other women through the journey of infertility.

Peer support and more helpful advice can be found on her website: *www.infaithility.com*

Acknowledgement

Firstly, I would like to thank and honour my God without whom I would have no story to tell.

I also acknowledge my publisher Daniella at Conscious Dreams Publishing, my editor Elise Abram and the amazing team that helped to bring my first book to life.

Works Cited

"A-Z Fertility Glossary: Intracytoplasmic Sperm Injection (ICSI)." *Human Fertilization & Embryology Authority*, www.hfea.gov.uk/treatments/explore-all-treatments/intracytoplasmic-sperm-injection-icsi/ Accessed 24 March 2024.

"A-Z Fertility Glossary: In vitro fertilisation (IVF)." *Human Fertilization & Embryology Authority*, www.hfea.gov.uk/about-us/a-z-fertility-glossary/#:~:text=In%20vitro%20fertilisation%20(IVF),woman's%20womb%20through%20the%20cervix. Accessed 14 March 2024.

"And Me: My Sperm Donor and Me." *BBC iPlayer*, 29 September 2023, https://www.bbc.co.uk/iplayer/episode/p0ggqtv3/and-me-my-sperm-donor-and-me. Accessed 14 March 2024.

Ali, Sumera et al. "Knowledge, perceptions and myths regarding infertility among selected adult population in Pakistan: a cross-sectional study." *BMC Public Health*, vol. 11, no. 760, 2011. *PubMed*, doi: 10.1186/1471-2458-11-760. Accessed 21 March 2024.

Arbo, Matthew. *Walking through Infertility: Biblical, Theological, And Moral Counsel for Those Who Are Struggling*. Crossway, 2018.

Bible: *The New King James Version*. Thomas Nelson, 2022.

Biga, Lindsay. M. et al. "28.2 Embryonic Development." *Anatomy and Physiology*, Openstax/Oregon State University, 2019. https://open.oregonstate.education/aandp/chapter/28-2-embryonic-development/. Accessed 09 April 2024.

Biga, Lindsay M. et al. "Anatomy & Physiology." *Oregon State University*, 2019, https://open.oregonstate.education/aandp/chapter/28-2-embryonic-development/. Accessed 14 March 2024.

Bulletti, Carlo, et al. "Progesterone: The Key Factor of the Beginning of Life." *International Journal of Molecular Sciences*, vol. 23, no. 22, 2022. *MDPI*, doi: 10.3390/ijms232214138.

Capps, Charles. *Faith and Confession*. Harrison House, 1987.

"Confidence." *Cambridge Dictionary*, https://dictionary.cambridge.org/dictionary/english/confidence. Accessed 14 March 2024.

DeCenso, Frank A., Jr. *Hearing and Understanding the Voice of God*. Destiny Image, 2011.

Elwell, Kristan. "The social and cultural consequences of infertility in rural and Peri-Urban Malawi." *African Journal of Reproductive Health*, vol. 26, no.7, 1 July 2022, pp. 112–126. *PubMed*, doi: 10.29063/ajrh2022/v26i7.3. Accessed 21 March 2024.

"Ethics of In Vitro Fertilization." *The Ethics Centre*, 8 April 2019, https://ethics.org.au/the-ethics-of-in-vitro-fertilization-ivf/. Accessed 14 March 2024.

"Ethnic diversity in fertility treatment 2018." *Human Fertilisation & Embryology Authority*, March 2021, https://www.hfea.gov.uk/about-us/publications/research-and-data/ethnic-diversity-in-fertility-treatment-2018/. Accessed 14 March 2024.

"Fear." *Cambridge Dictionary*, https://dictionary.cambridge.org/dictionary/english/fear. Accessed 14 March 2024.

Fleming, LaKeisha. "Egg Quality: What You Need to Know." *Very Well Family*, 26 August 2022, https://www.verywellfamily.com/how-to-support-egg-quality-5219743. Accessed 14 March 2024.

"Freedom Series Part 1." *YouTube*, uploaded by Brad Norman, 1 May 2022, https://www.youtube.com/watch?v=Dupfd28XojQ.

"Freedom Series Part 2." *YouTube*, uploaded by Brad Norman, 15 May 2022, https://www.youtube.com/watch?v=-vLu7tNMQeo.

"Girl, Get Up." *YouTube*, uploaded by Sarah Jakes-Roberts, 11 December 2019, https://www.youtube.com/watch?v=k3k8VEN13a0.

Johnson, Loree. "Infertility Trauma is Racial Trauma. And Implications for Where the Two Meet." *Thrive Global*, 06 June 2020, https://community.thriveglobal.com/infertility-trauma-is-racial-trauma/. Accessed 04 April 2024.

"Kellogg's to give staff fertility, menopause and miscarriage leave." *BBC*, 29 October 2021, https://www.bbc.com/news/uk-england-manchester-59089645. Accessed 14 March 2024.

Lamb, Sheila and Yemi Adegbile. *Infertility doesn't not care about your ethnicity, Heartbreaking and inspiring stories about infertility, IVF, miscarriage, and loss.* MFS Books Ltd., 2021.

Latham, Katherine. "How pollution is causing a male fertility crisis." *BBC*, 27 March 2023, https://www.bbc.com/future/article/20230327-how-pollution-is-causing-a-male-fertility-crisis. Accessed 14 March 2024.

Logan, Shanna, et al. "Infertility in China: Culture, society and a need for fertility counselling." *Asian Pacific Journal of Reproduction*, vol. 8, no.1, 2019, pp.1-6. *Research Gate*, doi:10.4103/2305-0500.250416. Accessed 21 March 2023.

Martins, Noni. *Unfertility.* https://unfertility.com/. Accessed 14 March 2024.

— "As an informed and evolved young Black woman, with exposure to information, even I blamed myself for our infertility." *Human Fertilisation & Embryology Authority*, 27 October 2020, https://www.hfea.gov.uk/about-us/our-blog/as-an-informed-and-evolved-young-black-woman-with-exposure-to-information-even-i-blamed-myself-for-our-infertility/. Accessed 14 March 2024.

Meyer, Joyce. *Battlefield of the Mind: Winning the Battle in Your Mind.* Word Alive, 2002.

"Modernizing fertility law." *Fertilisation & Embryology Authority*, November 2023, https://www.hfea.gov.uk/about-us/modernising-the-regulation-of-fertility-treatment-and-research-involving-human-embryos/modernising-fertility-law/. Accessed 14 March 2024.

"My Shock at discovering I was a donor child." *BBC*, 30 November 2017, https://www.bbc.co.uk/news/stories-42159574. Accessed 14 March 2024.

Osei, Thelma. "Why We Need to Talk About Racial Disparities in Fertility Care." *Illume Fertility*, 5 February 2024, https://www.illumefertility.com/fertility-blog/why-we-need-to-talk-about-racial-disparities-in-fertility-care. Accessed 14 March 2024.

"Overview: Ectopic pregnancy." *National Health Service*, 23 August 2022, https://www.nhs.uk/conditions/ectopic-pregnancy/. Accessed 14 March 2024.

"Overview: Fibroids." *National Health Service*, 9 September 2022, https://www.nhs.uk/conditions/fibroids/. Accessed 14 March 2024.

"Overview: Infertility." *National Health Service*, 9 August 2023, https://www.nhs.uk/conditions/infertility/. Accessed 14 March 2024.

Pashigian. Mellisa. J. "7. Conceiving the Happy family: Infertility and Marital Politics in Northern Vietnam." *Infertility around the Globe: New Thinking on Childlessness, Gender, and Reproductive Technologies*, edited by Marcia Inhorn and Frank van Balen, University of California Press, 2002, pp. 134-151.

"Royal Succession." *History*, 26 July 2017, https://www.history.com/topics/european-history/royal-succession. Accessed 14 March 2024.

Siddiqui, Aisha, et al. "Fetal Development: The 1st trimester." *Beacon Healthy System*, 3 June 2022, www.beaconhealthsystem.org/library/articles/fetal-development-the-1st-trimester?content_id=ART-20045302. Accessed 14 March 2024.

Strong, Carson. *Ethics in reproductive and perinatal medicine: A new framework*. Yale University, 2017.

van Rooij, Floor B., et al. "The experiences of involuntarily childless Turkish immigrants in the Netherlands." *Qualitative Health Research* vol. 19, no.5, 2009, pp 621–632. *Sage Journals*, doi:10.1177/1049732309333242.

Warren, Rick. *The Purpose Driven Life. What on earth am I here for?* Zondervan, 2013.

"Week 3." *Nemours Kids Health*, 2022, https://kidshealth.org/en/parents/week3.html. Accesssed 14 March 2024.

"What is the difference between a Day 3 and a Day 5 Embryo Transfer?" *San Diego Fertility Center Miracle Blog*, 2 September 2011, https://www.sdfertility.com/blog/what-is-the-difference-between-a-day-3-and-a-day-5-embryo-transfer. Accessed 14 March 2024.

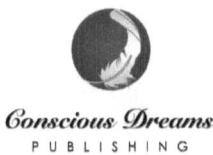

Conscious Dreams
PUBLISHING

Transforming diverse writers
into successful published authors

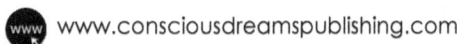 www.consciousdreamspublishing.com

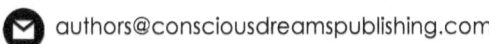 authors@consciousdreamspublishing.com

Let's connect

www.ingramcontent.com/pod-product-compliance
Lightning Source LLC
Chambersburg PA
CBHW030041100526
44590CB00011B/291